LANGUAGE DISORDERS IN SCHOOL-AGE CHILDREN

REMEDIATION OF COMMUNICATION DISORDERS SERIES
Frederick N. Martin, Series Editor

STUTTERING

———————————————————————— *Edward G. Conture*

HEARING IMPAIRMENTS IN YOUNG CHILDREN

———————————————————————— *Arthur Boothroyd*

HARD OF HEARING CHILDREN IN REGULAR SCHOOLS

Mark Ross with Diane Brackett
——————————————————— *and Antonia Maxon*

HEARING-HANDICAPPED ADULTS

———————————————————————— *Thomas G. Giolas*

ACQUIRED NEUROGENIC DISORDERS

———————————————————————— *Thomas P. Marquardt*

LANGUAGE DISORDERS IN PRESCHOOL CHILDREN

———————————————————————— *Patricia R. Cole*

LANGUAGE DISORDERS IN SCHOOL AGE CHILDREN

———————————————————————— *Mary Lovey Wood*

Forthcoming

ARTICULATION DISORDERS

———————————————————————— *Ronald K. Sommers*

CEREBRAL PALSY

———————————————————————— *James C. Hardy*

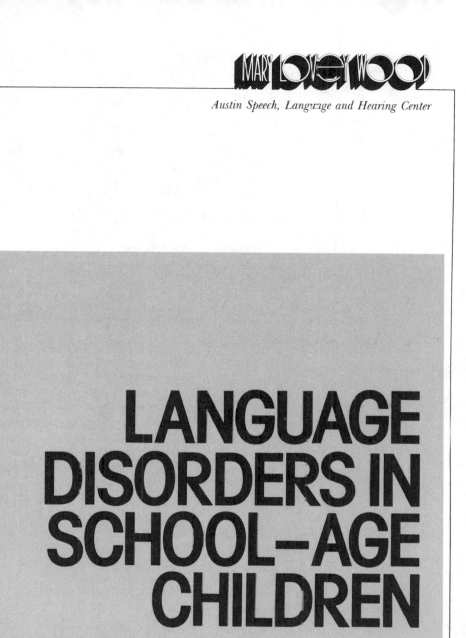

LANGUAGE DISORDERS IN SCHOOL–AGE CHILDREN

Prentice-Hall, Inc., Englewood Cliffs, New Jersey 07632

Library of Congress Cataloging in Publication Data

Wood, Mary Lovey.
    Language disorders in school-age children.
    (Remediation of communication disorders)
    Bibliography: p.
    Includes index.
    1. Language disorders in children. I. Title.
II. Series.
RJ496.L35W66   618.92'855   81-22723
ISBN 0-13-522946-4   AACR2

© 1982 by Prentice-Hall, Inc., Englewood Cliffs, N.J. 07632

Printed in the United States of America

10 9 8 7 6 5 4 3 2

Editorial production/supervision by Virginia Cavanagh Neri
Interior design by Maureen Olsen
Cover design by Maureen Olsen
Manufacturing buyer: Edmund W. Leone

ISBN 0-13-522946-4

Prentice-Hall International, Inc., *London*
Prentice-Hall of Australia Pty. Limited, *Sydney*
Prentice-Hall of Canada, Ltd., *Toronto*
Prentice-Hall of India Private Limited, *New Delhi*
Prentice-Hall of Japan, Inc., *Tokyo*
Prentice-Hall of Southeast Asia Pte. Ltd., *Singapore*
Whitehall Books Limited, *Wellington, New Zealand*

To all the children who have tried to teach me

#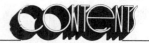

Introduction   1

Identification and assessment   12

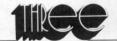

Intervention   85

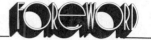

FOREWORD

With the information explosion of recent years there has been a proliferation of knowledge in the areas of scientific and social inquiry. The speciality of communicative disorders has been no exception. While two decades ago a single textbook or "handbook" might have sufficed to provide the aspiring or practicing clinician with enlightenment on an array of communication handicaps, this is no longer possible—hence the decision to prepare a series of single-author texts.

As the title implies, the emphasis of this series, *Remediation of Communication Disorders,* is on therapy and treatment. The authors of each book were asked to provide information relative to anatomical and physiological aspects of each disorder, as well as pathology, etiology, and diagnosis to the extent that an understanding of these factors bears on management procedures. In such relatively short books this was quite a challenge: to offer guidance without writing a "cookbook"; to be selective without being parochial; to offer theory without losing sight of practice. To this challenge the series' authors have risen magnificently.

Mary Lovey Wood has practiced in the field of speech and language remediation for more than sixteen years, the last ten of which have seen her specialize in children with spoken and written communication disorders. The reader will recognize that this is a book written by a practicing clinician who sees literally hundreds of language-impaired children each month. Dr. Wood's book is unique in that it offers theoretical bases for intervention along with specific suggestions for direct work on communication disorders of school-age children. This book provides specific guidelines for parents and teachers in the management of language-impaired children, and it provides special ways of interacting with tutors, psychologists, and sensory integration specialists in the cooperative treatment of these very special children. Dr. Wood is above all a humanist, whose sensitivity and dedication are apparent in this book.

FREDERICK N. MARTIN
Series Editor

"My mother took me and my sister."
"Took you where?"
"Yeah.'
"Your mother took you and your sister *where?*"
"Yes, she did. That will be the last one I'd ever seen."

The linguistic shock one can experience from conversing with a language-impaired individual can be as frustrating as it is amusing, depending on one's investment in the outcome of the conversation. Those of us who intervene with language-impaired children have a very large investment in the outcome, and we often fail to be amused. Slow changes in the child's language abilities, frustrated parents, and impatient teachers may minimize a clinician's effectiveness (to say nothing of one's reputation).

No one really cares what we "do" with language-impaired children—as long as it works. When it does work, we don't even have to pronounce it correctly. If intervention does not seem to be working, then we must explain what is being "done." This book is written with the intention of suggesting a few things that might work, or, in some instances, some things that might have been "done."

The help of numerous language-impaired children and their parents have gone into the writing of this book. (Some critics of the book have suggested that the children literally did the writing.) Many of my teachers and colleagues also are responsible for the philosophies reflected in the book. Specifically, I want to thank Dr. Alice Richardson, Ms. Martha McGlothlin, and Dr. Patricia Cole for their valuable assistance with the content and organization. Special thanks go to "The Psychologist," Dr. Marjorie Menefee; "The Sensory Integration Specialist," Ms. Pat Ramm; and "The Tutor," Ms. Jill Graham. My sincere appreciation to every clinician who tries to find what works—and keeps trying.

MARY LOVEY WOOD

LANGUAGE DISORDERS IN SCHOOL−AGE CHILDREN

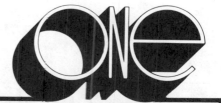

Introduction

Language-learning disorders do not begin or disappear with enrollment in kindergarten or first grade, and their effects may continue into adulthood. As a child matures, an oral language impairment may become less obvious to the casual listener but still interfere with classroom behavior and social functioning. In many school-age children, language deviations and poor academic achievement are the residual effects of earlier language disorders. In some school-age children, academic difficulty and behavior problems are the first observed evidence of inadequate language skills.

Late identification of language deficiencies complicates the consideration of intervention and can lead to parental confusion and professional buck-passing. Teachers may hesitate to report problems because they fear admonishment from parents or administrators for not coping better with a difficult child. Parents may not have suspected learning problems before the child entered school, although they may have harboured anxieties about certain aspects of behavior or development. If the child's language disorder was diagnosed prior to school age, new problems of classroom and home management may emerge when the child enters school. Early intervention may have minimized the deficiency, but some of the problems remain and are aggravated because the school setting stresses an inadequate language system.

The child is expected to pay attention to one person in the midst of noise and distraction, to understand new information which is often spoken only once, and to respond to questions with appropriate answers. Requiring the child to use his/her oral language to learn an entirely new method of communicating in written form further escalates stress on an already burdened language system. Oral language skills, which may be barely adequate for listening and speaking to just one person, may fail the child who is trying to function under the pressure of classroom interaction. "The single most significant deterrent to educational growth remains the inability to use oral and written language, to speak and to read" (Stark and Wallach, 1980, p. 6). Preschool developmental inadequacies seem less important and less alarming than the same impairment measured in academic and social terms.

Language-impaired children themselves may not have to confront their problems in self-evaluative terms until they enter school, where their struggles take on added dimensions. They may find themselves inadequate in comparison to other children; classmates tease them and teachers reproach them. Children with language deficiencies may question their own abilities, thereby negatively influencing their feelings of self-worth (Wiig and Semel, 1976).

○ CAMOUFLAGE AND SIGNALS

It is unfortunate that so many forms of language deficiency are camouflaged until the child has shown many signs of failure or frustration. Unless the child talks like a telegram, omitting words and using gestures, a language disorder may remain undetected until the child reaches school. Many language-deficient children talk excessively and develop large vocabularies that hide problems in language processing and mask expressive deficiencies (Wiig and Semel, 1976). Early difficulty with preacademic skills such as identifying sounds by letter name, recognizing sound differences, and identifying letters, may indicate potential difficulty in using language to learn to read (*Asha,* 1980; Wiig and Semel, 1976, 1980). When the child enters first grade, the same difficulties may persist, although some children manage to survive the requirements of first-grade work by memorizing words and phrases for their reading performances. Unless the child's language problems are very mild, the deficits in word analysis, phonics, and use of language to learn new material in class are obvious by the second grade. By third and fourth grade the problems are interfering with achievement. Language production in both oral and written form is noticeably inadequate, affecting both reading comprehension and math skills (Wiig and Semel 1976, 1980).

Many language-impaired children become hopelessly lost trying to do fourth-grade work. Specific help on the mechanics of reading and writing have been eliminated from classroom work; greater demands are made of the child to receive and respond to semantic variations, logical processing, and implications of complex material. Inadequate language skills may also begin to take their toll on the child's social interactions in the higher grades. Inability to interpret hints or respond to the unstated intent of a message may interfere with the quality of interpersonal relationships experienced by the young adolescent with language impairment (Wiig and Semel, 1976; 1980). When the child enters junior and senior high school, demands increase to interpret abstract material, understand linguistic ambiguities, and relate previously learned information to new materials which must be self-taught.

It is no longer enough to consider language development in terms of stringing together words in increasingly more complicated utterances. Attention must be paid to the way in which meaning is signaled, the relationship among words, and the use of words, phrases, and sentences. Language-impaired children are no longer evaluated solely in terms of whether they can manipulate the language system of their community. They are also "evaluated in terms of their ability to manipulate that code to achieve their communicative purposes" (Snyder, 1980, p. 32). Language acquisition must be considered in terms of the development of communicative competence, which includes the following:

1. Understanding of linguistic rules, which enables appropriate comprehension of and production of utterances (encompassing phonological, syntactic, morphological, and semantic components of language)
2. Use of language in a social context (Rees, 1978; *Asha* 1980; Stark and Wallach, 1980)

○ COMMUNICATIVE COMPETENCE

Trends regarding language acquisition and remediation have moved from teaching children to talk to teaching children to communicate. Any clinician who has tried to improve language skills in language deficient children can appreciate a story related by Rees (1978, p. 193) describing the language skills of a child who had received traditional intervention designed to improve expressive language skills. The child was handed a cup and responded:

"It's a cup."

"It's pink."

"It's plastic."

"You drink out of it."

It is unlikely that this child could formulate a request for a drink of water when thirsty, but she could recite the sentences she had learned for describing a particular object.

In light of this example, Rees differentiates *communicative competence* from *linguistic competence.* She notes that the traditional definition of linguistic competence describes the ideal speaker's/hearer's knowledge of the rules that account for grammaticality of language. The child who responded to the cup in the foregoing example might be considered linguistically competent. In contrast, a definition of communicative competence would include a language user's knowledge of language as a "shared social system with rules for correct use in given contexts" (Rees, 1978, p. 194).

Many linguistic models of communication tend to ignore some fundamental facts about the way people communicate (Krause, 1979). Models of linguistic competence suggest that strings of definable structures, such as sounds, words, and word combinations, are produced and understood as representations of ideas. The implications are that the exchange of ideas is conducted by the strings of symbols alone and that the message exists separately from the linguistic or social context in which it occurs. Theories of communicative competence indicate that there is no necessary relationship between the strings of words used to convey a message and the intended meaning or effect. In addition to knowledge of the components of linguistic competence, such as content and form of language, the communicatively competent individual must also know how to use language in the context of social interaction. The use of language in social interaction includes the following variables:

1. Carrying on a conversation, including turn taking and responding to another's utterances
2. Communicating in a socially and situationally appropriate way, including attending to the listener's knowledge and relationship to the speaker (sex, age, familiarity)
3. Maintaining the topic of conversation
4. Organizing and directing behavior

We communicate in order to affect the behavior of others, and efforts to accomplish that feat include the interaction of numerous verbal and nonverbal components.

the problem and the territory

As our understanding of communication expands, so does our realization of the complexities and subtleties of diagnosing and intervening with communication deficits. The intricacies of communication disorders often lead to categorizing components of language for the sake of easier assessment and intervention planning. However, a move toward sectionizing parts of communication may not be productive. Wallach and Lee note that overcompartmentalizing language may "lead professionals to devise tasks contrary to the way oral and written language actually develops" (Wallach and Lee, 1980, p. 100).

The political battles that are fought to separate language disorders from learning disorders appear foolish when one considers the impact of language on all aspects of learning. For example, The Education of the Handicapped Act, (PL 94–142) defines a specific learning disability as a disorder in one or more of the basic psychological processes involved in understanding or using language, spoken or written, which may manifest itself in an imperfect ability to listen, think, speak, read, write, spell, or do mathematical calculations. The federal regulation (1977) indicates that an individual may have a specific learning disability when there is a severe discrepancy between achievement and intellectual ability in one or more of the following areas:

1. Oral expression
2. Listening comprehension
3. Written expression
4. Basic reading skill
5. Reading comprehension
6. Mathematical calculation
7. Mathematical reasoning

It seems apparent that a person with a language disability could experience interference in one or more of these areas in spite of adequate intellectual potential (*Asha,* 1975, 1980; Stark and Wallach, 1980). It is not possible to separate language disabilities from learning disabilities in a clear-cut way because of the influence of language on all aspects of learning and functioning.

Richardson noted the identification of two major categories of learning disabled: (1) children whose school failure is in reading and spelling, and (2) children whose school problems are more generalized and include arithmetic (Richardson, 1976, p. iii). Richardson indicated that those with reading disability tend to score higher on performance items on standardized assessment measures and show specific problems in establishing verbal associations. The second group tends to demonstrate perceptual motor deficits. The two groups are not mutually exclusive, however, and frequently we see children with difficulties in all aspects of schoolwork as well as in social interaction.

Traditionally, a school system has assumed that a child enters school with adequate language skills. Some children do not have intact language systems when they enter school, while others fail to develop the necessary language competencies in listening, speaking, reading, and writing after beginning school (*Asha,* 1980). Since language underlies the major portion of academic learning, it cannot be separated from instruction or the curriculum. "It seems apparent . . . that one cannot separate reading from language itself . . . nor . . . clearly separate reading disabilities from language disabilities from learning disabilities" (Richardson, 1976, iii). Arbitrary separation of spoken from written language interferes with the designing of intervention programs for language disabled children (*Asha,* 1975, 1980; Bryan, 1978).

Reading is only incidental to the development of language comprehension and cognitive ability; a description of reading comprehension has to be a description of language comprehension (Carroll, 1977). The integration of semantic and syntactic clues is essential to good reading. Current trends indicate an awareness of cognitive and linguistic deficits in children with learning disabilities and the relationship of these deficits to reading difficulties (Vogel, 1974; Wiig and Semel, 1975; Snyder, 1980; Vellutino, 1978).

Other subjects that appear to be nonlanguage based, such as mathematics, can no longer be considered outside the realm of the language specialist. Mathematics includes more than numerical operations; it "requires a basic language and conceptual repertoire as prerequisites for the development of abstractions necessary for problem solving" (Carlson, Gruenewald, and Nyberg, 1980, p. 60). Solving verbal mathematical problems requires the use of language skills to determine the necessary problem-solving operation (Wiig and Semel, 1980). Although science is based largely in spatial or visual experiences, language proficiencies are necessary for the child to understand certain concepts, particularly if those concepts are space and time related (Wiig and Semel, 1980).

In spite of the deluge of information regarding language assessment, communicative competence, and learning disorders, teachers and clinicians have difficulty integrating this information with intervention and curriculum. One reason may be that the various aspects of language and learning, such as mathematics tutoring, remedial reading, language therapy, and spelling drills, are treated as separate entities (Carlson, Gruenewald, and Nyberg, 1980). Because language disorders disrupt so many parts of the child's school and home life, intervention *must* involve the coordinated efforts of the key people in the child's life.

intervention

The commitment to intervene with language-impaired children includes much more than providing technical assistance to change mistakes in speech (or comprehension, or reading, or spelling, or classroom behavior). Intervention involves long-term efforts with the child, the family, and the many other professionals who may be consulted for assistance. Coordination of efforts to help the child is part of the responsibility of the remediation specialist. This specialist, whether teacher, resource teacher, psychologist, tutor, or speech-language clinician, must provide support and advice to the child's parents as they seek appropriate help. Even the most capable parents do not know what resources are available, what questions to ask, or what requests to make on their child's behalf. Too often the major concern of the remediation specialist is limited to the content of his/her work with the child.

The quality of the intervention process is the key to improving communicative competence. Materials and tasks tend to be oriented toward skill building, but language is not a splinter skill or solely a group of skills. Because the intervention process encompasses everything from coordinating the help the child receives to long-term direct contact with the child, the quality of intervention is more affected by what the clinician does with content and tasks than his/her choice of materials and goals The process

of intervention for the development of communicative competence should
include these essentials:

> *Facilitating active learning so the child has access to abilities not previously
> available.* This can be compared to a traditional approach to teaching in which
> information is presented and drills are set up to achieve performance goals.
> In the traditional approach to intervention, a child usually is considered an
> object for change as the teacher sees fit. The active learning approach is more
> effective because the child learns to consider and use new language behav-
> iors in communication events of personal importance. The clinician must
> attend to the child's use of language in communication and adapt the interven-
> tion content to the child. Prescriptive teaching methods and prepackaged kits
> for skill building rarely provide an opportunity for communication within the
> structured teaching/learning situation.

> *Allowing for the establishment and application of rule-governed behaviors,
> rather than limited and memorized tasks.* The clinician must consider lan-
> guage a tool for communication and learning, not a static product.

> *Providing intervention services by a specialist knowledgeable in the form,
> content, and use of normal and deficient language.* The specialist must attend
> to the effect of language behavior on the child's academic and personal
> functioning and intervene appropriately. Good intentions and a kind heart are
> not sufficient for improving communicative competence.

Regardless of the severity of the language disorder, the time the problem
was identified or whether optimum intervention is provided, school-age
children with language learning deficiencies present enormous obstacles for
all who encounter them. Intervention should minimize these obstacles for
children and their parents and teachers.

○ SCOPE AND PURPOSE OF THE BOOK

This book discusses various forms of communication disorders in
school-age children and adolescents and suggests appropriate intervention
approaches. Chapter Two discusses individual differences among language-
deficient children, emphasizing the need to consider the interaction of all
components of the language system in the indentification and assessment
processes. Frequently, multiple means of assessing communication behaviors are necessary, and relying solely on quantitative standardized tests may
be inadequate for obtaining complete evaluation data. Nonstandardized,
criterion-referenced procedures often provide valuable information on language and communication performance.

Chapter Two also examines identification procedures for language impairment and provides guidelines for screening school-age children. Assessment of communication behaviors is described in terms of deviations
of the language system, expressive deficiencies, receptive deficiencies, and

organizational deficiencies. The components of expressive and receptive deficiencies are identified and discussed as aspects of language—use, content, and form—along with qualitative and quantitative assessment procedures for each. Disorders often associated with, or accompanying, communication deficiencies include problems in social behaviors, difficulty with selective attention, and general disorganization of actions and life activities. Written language disorders, such as problems with reading, spelling, or writing, frequently occur in children with oral language deficits. Chapter Two looks at the requirements written language places on the language-impaired child and suggests procedures for identifying deficiencies.

Chapter Three discusses indirect intervention, including the use of referrals and resources, and direct intervention. Numerous examples from clinical experience illustrate aspects of the intervention process. Suggestions for classroom and home management of language-deficient children are not intended to be prescriptive. Each child presents a unique and constantly changing set of problems; no child ever fits neatly into a diagnostic category or label. Suggestions are intended only to illustrate and serve as general approaches for creating and executing intervention plans. The book concludes with a discussion of the process of intervention and the expertise required of the intervention specialist.

The contents of this book are particularly applicable to school-age children and adolescents with near-average or above-average intellectual potential and a pattern of specific deficiencies in the learning or use of their native language. Special adaptations of the material would be necessary for students with sensory or orthopedic impairments, and many sections of the book are not appropriate for children with global retardation or severe sensory/physical impairments. This material is for the specialist in communication disorders, although some sections might be useful to other specialists, teachers, and parents.

Approaches to language intervention presented here emphasize the integration of language form and content with language use. In order to emphasize communicative competence and not just language competence in the intervention process, components of use are stressed rather than components of form and content. Numerous sources in the literature describe assessment and remediation approaches for disorders of form and content, often ignoring the use to which language is put, both interpersonally and intrapersonally. Children learn language through its use, and then they acquire the necessary content and form for receiving and conveying the linguistic complexities of communication. The use of language as a tool for interaction and as a device for learning is the core of communication and the intended emphasis of this book.

Because of the number of different terms applied to children without adequate language, and because of the lack of universally accepted definitions of terms, it is necessary to define elements of frequently used words that appear in the following discussions.

○ DEFINITIONS

Communicative competence represents the speaker's ability to effectively communicate an intentional message in order to alter the listener's attitudes, beliefs, and/or behaviors (Lucas, 1980). Hymes (1972) defined communicative competence as what the language user knows about who can say what in what ways, when, and where, and to whom. The communication process involves the exchange of ideas, intentions, or information among individuals and may occur through the application of verbal or nonverbal means (Wiig and Semel, 1976). Communicative competence requires the integration of the components of the language system—of use, content, and form (Bloom and Lahey, 1978).

Language use, called the pragmatics of language, encompasses the way in which *structure* of utterances and *content* of words and word combinations are applied for communicative interaction, intrapersonal development, and learning. A pragmatic approach to language involves studies of language use in social context and discourse, including the ability to produce or understand utterances that are contextually appropriate (Rees, 1978). Pragmatics includes the use of the language components of structure and content to convey an intended message. The study of language use, or pragmatics, can be categorized into: (1) the intention of communication for communicative interaction, and (2) language competencies of content, form, and interactive devices for learning and for personal growth.

Linguistic competence denotes the ideal speaker's/hearer's knowledge of rules for producing and understanding grammatical structures (form) that are meaningfully appropriate (content) (Rees, 1978; Lucas, 1980). *Content* is the represented information or meaning in a message, within the utterance or series of utterances, and includes compositional and referential aspects. Content is sometimes referred to as *semantics* and includes the study of the relationships between words and grammatical forms and their underlying meanings (Wiig and Semel, 1976). The *form* or structure of language refers to the phonological rules, the syntactical rules, and the morphological rules in the reception and production of utterances. A discussion of *phonology,* the sound system of language, is not included in this material. *Syntax* specifies word order of utterances. *Morphology* refers to the study of the smallest unit of meaning in language. Grammatical morphemes can be classified as either free or bound, depending on whether or not they occur in isolation, such as prepositions (in, on), or inflections on words (cat*s*).

The term *language impairment* represents the presence of specific deficiencies in the symbol system of the native language. Terms that are used interchangeably to denote inadequacies in components of use, content, or form of the oral or written symbol system include: *language deviation, language disability, language-learning impairment, language disorder,* and *language dysfunction.*

The analysis of language disorders and attempts at remediation are demanding tasks. Solutions to the problems posed by inadequate language are as evasive as the attention of language-impaired children. This dilemma requires continued efforts in the face of frustration because sometimes we succeed. The more we attempt to teach the children, the more they can teach us.

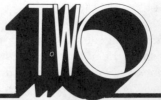

Identification and assessment

Assessing and describing children with language disorders are particularly difficult because the range and variety of problems prevent easy labeling or categorization. As Stark and Wallach (1980) point out, the imprecision in diagnostic categories and the complexity of the categorization process lead many diagnosticians to conclude that describing behaviors is more useful than labeling them. Each language-deficient child differs from every other in the ways he/she receives information, expresses himself/herself, and interacts with other people. However, many language-deficient children possess common characteristics in their interaction with other people. It seems that language-impaired children live within their own experiential world, perceiving and responding to experiences through a unique set of filters. Events and situations interpreted through inadequate language systems may become distortions of time, space, sound, and interaction. Some language-deficient children and adolescents talk and act as though they are not quite tuned in to the rest of the world.

○ INDIVIDUAL DIFFERENCES IN LANGUAGE-DEFICIENT CHILDREN

The search for similarities among various language-impaired children sometimes minimizes the importance of individual differences among them. The ways in which language-impaired children are identified and described for analysis as well as for intervention are important in assessing the linguistic characteristics of the language impairment. Aram and Nation (1975, p. 230) indicated that grouping any children with language disorders into one category, or grouping by etiology, "obscures linguistic differences presented by the children." Quantitative descriptions of language-impaired children are complicated and even contaminated by the normalizing effects of statistical treatment of means. Most studies group language-impaired children for statistical treatment rather than describing and analyzing their utterances qualitatively. Complete analysis of aspects of language samples frequently is considered too large a task; therefore, many distinctions are ignored and different patterns are lumped together in a single category to reduce the number of categories that must be listed and tabulated. The distinction ignored in one study may be the distinction of principal interest in the next.

Some studies emphasize the quantitative evaluation of deviant language, minimizing the qualitative information for the sake of counting frequency of structure types used. Those studies often report results that are quantitative in nature because the questions asked in the study require treatment of numerical data. The relationship among language subsystems (for example, from semantics to morphology) or within subsystems (for example, types of grammatical errors) or among individual subjects (for example, differences in types of language disorders represented within a group) are not always considered.

Another form of quantitative analysis which may smooth out qualitative differences is that of grouping and averaging. The treatment of averaging on groups of diverse individuals does not provide descriptive information about individuals within the groups, and the conclusions should not imply that it does. For example, in some studies, children are grouped and the performances of each group are averaged. (Morehead and Ingram, 1973). It is possible in such studies that some of the language-impaired children produced none of the linguistic forms and some produced all of the structures, yielding an average of 50 percent for the group. This score is meaningless in many studies, particularly if errors and distortions made by the various children are not described. Group data may not indicate that individual deviations within the group suggest great variability from child to child.

Some linguistically-deviant children convey complex intentions through high-level sentence construction with embedding and coordination. For example, "I don't know he be on yet," would be interpreted as "I don't know if he has been on yet." "In water try them, get that with them fishing pole" would be interpreted as "In the water, they tried to get that fish with their fishing pole." However, the use of morphemes and verb constructions may be extremely limited. If number of morphemes per utterance were used to determine linguistic level, (Morehead and Ingram, 1973), some linguistically deviant children would fall within the lower linguistic levels. If semantic constituents or relationships were used to determine linguistic level, the same linguistically deviant child might fall within the higher levels. When different components are considered for each child, it is apparent that some children are not developing language skills in an orderly, progressive manner. One child might be grouped in a research project with another child who has different linguistic deviations; an average of their performances might be traceable on a developmental scale, but not reflective of either child's language behavior.

Counting errors in one linguistic component in isolation from errors in another part of the system may not reveal deviations in language acquisition. Failure to uncover qualitative differences between the language-deviant and the normal child may result in the opinion that there are no qualitative differences between linguistically-deviant children and normal-speaking children.

Research methods, evaluation tools, and intervention programs often reflect assumptions that may mask such important linguistic deviations as

> Making generalizations from frequency counts in averaged responses of heterogeneously grouped children
>
> Failing to compare components within the child's language system (for example, comparing structural development with semantic development)

With individualized qualitative analysis of language, assessment and intervention may avoid oversimplifying the complexities of communication. The clinician must interpret group data with caution, taking care to analyze within-group variance.

analysis of communication

The complexities of communication lead the language specialist on a continuing search for effective ways of assessing and remediating language deficiencies. Traditional approaches to language analysis have dealt with the structural analysis of grammar and phonology, including descriptions of sound production, syntax, and grammatical constructions (Travis, 1957; Van Riper, 1962; Lee, 1969; Lee and Canter, 1971). Early psycholinguistic approaches incorporated modality performances such as input, association, memory and sequencing (Kirk, McCarthy, and Kirk, 1968). More recent attention has been focused on the semantic components of communication (Fillmore, 1968; Chafe, 1970; Brown, 1973). Many current language specialists feel that language use and not form or content should comprise the basis of language training (Muma, 1978; Rees, 1978). In whatever way language is analyzed, it must be regarded within its communicative context and as a system of integrated parts.

language as a system of integrated parts

Since the early 1970s, language studies have recognized the interaction of pragmatic, semantic, and syntactic knowledge that children possess. Carol Chomsky (1969) indicates that children possess implicit linguistic knowledge and demonstrate that knowledge in assigning interpretations to the structures presented to them. Interpretation of grammatical rules affects the meaning children assign to utterances. Jackendorf (1972) provides an overview of semantics and the impact of semantics on overt syntactic patterns of English. He discusses the theory of generative semantics, which asserts that syntax and semantics are inseparable and homogeneous in the normal speaker. The semantic interpretation of a sentence is considered a composite of various items of information about meaning and structure.

Wiig and Semel (1980) note the complexity of language by discussing a number of mental and language skills required for production of an appropriate message. These skills include choosing the vocabulary and syntactic structure to convey the ideas, matching the appropriate sounds to the words, and organizing the words to encode the intended meaning with the appropriate structure. The integration of form, content, and use is required for the proper selection of words and utterance forms to convey the intended message in a socially appropriate manner. For example, the intent of the message can be conveyed with different forms and choices of words depending on the situation:

> "Close the *#! door right now!"
>
> "Please close the door."
>
> "Does the room seem too cool with the door open?"

The entire process of producing an appropriate message occurs very rapidly in the normal speaker, with errors noted and corrected immediately. Many normal-speaking children understand and produce very complex messages before school-age. When children do not understand and use the complexities of communication, the remediation specialist must analyze and attend to the deficiencies. Children present an endless variety of ways to speak or write inadequately. A simple description of normal or deficient language cannot account for all the communicative deviations language-impaired children exhibit. Recognizing an existing language disorder can be fairly simple if the child shows overt signs of speech problems, such as misarticulations, poor sentence construction, or comprehension problems. A more difficult task is identifying a communication disorder when the child's speech is not obviously affected, at least to the ear of the casual listener.

○ IDENTIFICATION OF COMMUNICATION DISORDERS

Identification of communication disorders often occurs before the communication specialist even sees a child for confirmation and analysis of the problem. Parents, day-care workers, preschool and school teachers, audiologists, physicians, psychologists, and tutors may have the first opportunity to identify a communication problem. In some situations the communication specialist has a chance to provide screening services to preschool and school classes. In any of these instances, it is important for the observer to have some reliable guidelines for determining the presence or absence of a communication disorder. The greatest error made in the process of screening is overlooking a child's deficits by attributing the problems to "immaturity" or "poor work habits," particularly if a child's parent or teacher has expressed concerns about the child's functioning. Concern about a child's development by a parent or teacher is in itself a good screening device and is an adequate reason for referral for assessment.

formal screening instruments

Although many screening devices involve non-standardized observations, a few formal screening measures are now available. Two of the screening tests are by Semel and Wiig (1980) and compose parts of a more complete evaluation battery called the *Clinical Evaluation of Language Function (CELF)*. One of them, Elementary Screening for Kindergarten through 5th Grade, includes receptive-language and expressive-language screening items and takes approximately fifteen minutes to administer. The other is the Advanced Level Screening for Fifth through Twelfth Grade.

Another screening tool, the *Screening Test of Adolescent Language,* is by Prager, Beecher, Stafford, and Wallace (1980). The STAL is designed to identify students who appear sufficiently deviant in specific linguistic skills to require further testing. The screening test is divided into four categories —vocabulary, auditory memory span, language processing, and proverb explanation. Administration takes about ten minutes and cut-off scores are provided for grades six through eight and nine through twelve.

The *Stephens Oral Language Screening Test (SOLST)* (1977) is designed to screen for problems in expressive syntax and articulation in children ranging from four and one-half to seven years old. The test is a sentence-repetition task with sentences varying in length and complexity of construction. Administration time is approximately four minutes. Cut-off scores for each age level provide indicators of the need for further evaluation.

informal screening devices

School-age language-impaired children often are identified first by social problems or poor school achievement; these may be difficulties directly related to language disorders but not recognized as such. The most-commonly identified problems in school-age children with language deficiencies include:

1. Inadequacies in social behavior
2. Problems in memory and attention

3. Poor organization and self-direction
4. Poor academic achievement, particularly in reading and spelling

It is not unusual for a child with problems in one area, such as spoken language, to have difficulty in another area, such as school achievement.

The assessing clinician must exercise restraint against the temptation to cease the assessment procedure once a problem has been described. Since many children with deficits in one area do have problems in another area, the clinician's responsibility includes the continued evaluation of a child until all possible aspects of learning and functioning have been considered.

Age-related or grade-related guidelines for observation can be helpful when considering a child for complete evaluation and when formal screening is not desired. Cole and Wood (1978) describe some characteristics of various oral language deficiencies and related behaviors. Their outline (see figure 2–1) includes a list of both test behaviors and everyday behaviors of school-age children with oral language deficiencies. It is not intended to be exhaustive, and not all language-impaired children will display all the behaviors listed.

The authors suggest that any child demonstrating combinations of the outlined characteristics should be considered for complete assessment.

The purpose of this screening device, as with most other screening instruments, is to provide a framework for observing numerous facets of behavior that may deviate from acceptable ranges of functioning. For example, a child with adequate hearing who exhibits an impairment in understanding auditory information may respond to speech as if he/she had a hearing loss. Some children do not respond to speech at all in the presence of noise. In fact, they may object strenuously to background noise ("Turn off the vacuum. It hurts my ears."). Some children with deficiencies in auditory reception/comprehension do not answer utterances addressed to them but merely "echo" or imitate the utterance. Others, who understand words if they are accompanied by gestures or pictures, do not understand words without such nonverbal aids.

Children with milder versions of auditory receptive disorders may have difficulty understanding messages in group situations, or they may not remember important information addressed to them, or they may not generalize one item of information to similar-but-not-identical situations. [Clinician: "The match is burning and it's hot. I'll light the candle and make the candle burn." (*demonstrates*) "Will the candle be hot?" Child: "No, I can touch it 'cause it's not a match."] Behaviors, as listed in the Cole and Wood outline, can be indicative of significant problems and serve as indicators of problems. Examples of problems in auditory reception, as well as verbal expression, social behaviors, and academic behaviors, will be discussed in more detail in following sections.

FIGURE 2-1 DIAGNOSTICALLY SIGNIFICANT BEHAVIORS OF CHILDREN WITH NONSEN-SORY AUDITORY DISORDERS Cole, P., and L. Wood, "Differential Diagnosis," in *Pediatric Audiology,* Ed. F. N. Martin, Englewood Cliffs, New Jersey. Prentice-Hall, Inc., 1978. Reprinted by permission.

I. Auditory Reception
   A. Disregard of speech or all sounds
   B. Better responses in quiet than in noise
   C. Hypersensitivity to sound
   D. Echolalia
   E. Difficulty following verbal instructions unless accompanied by visual demonstrations
   F. Difficulty learning in group situations
   G. Failure to remember what people say
   H. Failure to generalize information from one experience to another
II. Verbal Expression
   A. Reduced quantity of verbalization
   B. Inadequate vocabulary
   C. Defective sentence structure
   D. Inability to verbalize experiences using a series of utterances
   E. Incorrect pronunciation (articulation) of words
   F. Disorganized content within or among utterances
   G. Dependence on gestures to express information
   H. Unusually literal content in ideas expressed
III. Social-Emotional Behaviors
   A. Problems in attention to pertinent tasks
   B. Inability to inhibit behavior
   C. Inability to cope with change
   D. Disorientation in space and time
   E. Immature self-help skills
   F. Perseveration
   G. Hyperactivity
   H. Inappropriate emotional reactions
   I. Social isolation
   J. Extreme aggression
   K. Limited interpersonal relationships
IV. Academic Behaviors
   A. Difficulty following verbal instructions or learning from verbal explanations in the classroom
   B. Difficulty learning phonics
   C. Inadequate reading or spelling
   D. Poor comprehension of what is read
   E. Disorganization in content of written material
   F. Poor sentence construction in written work
   G. Discrepancy between achievement level and potential for learning
V. Test Behaviors
   A. Significant discrepancy between verbal and nonverbal scores
   B. Low scores on verbal tests
   C. Discrepancy between test-retest scores on same measure or on tests designed to measure similar abilities
   D. Low achievement test scores

Discrepancies between verbal and nonverbal items have been recognized as possible indicators of learning impairment. If a child performs well on a series of tests designed to measure visual-motor abilities and performs poorly in verbal tasks, then additional evaluation is indicated to confirm the suspicion of language impairment.

Another discrepancy in behavior not noted explicitly in the Cole and Wood outline is that between everyday classroom performance and test performance. Some older children with language disorders or related problems obtain high scores on achievement tests but receive failing grades in school. The language-impaired child may do well with the structures of time and activity that a formal test provides, but not perform as well in situations of independent study or with the looser boundaries of group work. On the other hand, some children who are slow readers are penalized on timed tests because they do not complete the required tasks but perform quite well in class when allowed to work at their own rate.

Additional screening guidelines for preschool and school-age children are intended to provide a framework for observing various aspects of children's behavior when considering additional evaluation (see Figures 2-2 and 2-3). Adapted from personal experience, they incorporate guidelines provided by other communication specialists (Johnson and Myklebust, 1967; Bangs, 1968, 1982; Lucas, 1980; Snyder, 1980; Stark and Wallach, 1980; Wiig and Semel, 1976, 1980).

FIGURE 2-2 SCREENING GUIDELINES FOR PRESCHOOL AND EARLY SCHOOL-AGE CHILDREN

1. Immature or babyish behavior
2. Difficulty learning preschool (readiness) tasks
   a. reciting or identifying letters of the alphabet
   b. reciting or identifying numbers under ten
   c. sound blending
   d. rhyming
   e. pronouncing long words (pinano/piano) or (aminal/animal)
   f. telling names of items within a semantic category
   g. difficulty matching sounds to letters (phonics)
3. Excessively hard to control
   a. inappropriately loud or unruly
   b. constantly active
4. Excessively passive and quiet
   a. minimal responses to questions
   b. noninitiation of conversations
   c. poor eye contact
5. Obvious difficulty with sound production, grammar, word combinations, or word use
6. Obvious difficulty with following directions, learning games, following classroom routine
7. Inconsistent behavior or learning, so that the child does some thing well one day, but acts noncomprehending of the task the next day
8. Alert and smart in some ways but very slow at learning in other ways

FIGURE 2–3 SCREENING GUIDELINES FOR SCHOOL-AGE CHILDREN AND ADOLESCENTS

1. Grammatical or organizational errors in oral and/or written language production, such as use of irregular plurals, verb tense, complex sentences, interpreting ambiguities or figurative forms of expression
2. Difficulty with aspects of written language, including sight reading and word-attack skills, spelling, interpreting the meaning of written material, quantity and quality of written work
3. Literal response to instructions or questions, although not appearing to understand that the response is inappropriate, or difficulty with implied cause-and-effect relationships
4. Good achievement scores combined with low classroom and homework performance, or poor test scores, with good classwork
5. Skill in one area (mathematics) and poor performance in another (reading and spelling)
6. Immaturity or silliness
7. Difficulty adhering to classroom rules and etiquette (speaking out of turn, bumping others out of the way, interrupting another child to answer, responding to the teacher without appropriate respect) although basically compliant
8. Excessive quietness and passivity
9. Excessive undirected activity
10. Disorganized or apparently irresponsible behavior, such as not doing homework assignments, losing lunch tickets, turning in incomplete work
11. Inconsistent behavior or learning, in that the child does not remember or apply previously learned information or skills
12. Poor recall or attention to new information or important detail
13. Tendency to cover up failure by cheating or lying about schoolwork

Loban (1963) provides an Oral Language Scale that collapses several dimensions of language use, content, and form into seven areas of observation for rating on a scale. The scale provides different ways to observe children's behaviors. With contrastive descriptive statements, the scale ranges from one to five and is summarized in the following polar positions:

1. *Skill in communication*
   shows no awareness of listeners   adjusts speech for listener
   (for example, makes no effort to
   evoke understanding from listeners)

2. *Organization, purpose, and control
   of language*
   rambles without purpose and   gets to the point and
   tells stories out of sequence   relates events in logical order

3. *Wealth of ideas*
   Seems dull and unimaginative   appears imaginative and creative

4. *Amount of language*
   seldom talks and needs to   talks frequently and freely
   be prompted

5. *Vocabulary*
   displays meager vocabulary   employs a rich variety of words

6. *Quality of listening*
   inattentive—rarely listens   shows excellent attentiveness
   to others   and responsiveness to speech of
                                       others

7. *Quality of language structure*
   uses simple sentences and omits   uses mature sentence patterns
   structural components   with phrases, clauses, and
                                       appropriate verb forms

The observer rates the child on the scale from 1 (lowest functioning) to 5 (highest functioning) on the basis of the child's communicative interactions. The ratings provide the observer with a means of judging a child's interactive communicative skills in conversational situations. Screening measures should not be used as the basis for judging developmental adequacy because they are often only gross measurements of skills and usually isolate separate aspects of behavior. The use of screening devices does provide the observer with structure and procedure for identifying children for complete assessment.

○ ASSESSMENT OF COMMUNICATION DISORDERS

Identification and analysis of communication disorders require the recognition of patterns of deficient behaviors. Standardized tests do not always indicate deficient language and learning patterns, and the appropriate interpretation of data can be difficult. The clinician must use any conceivable devices to obtain information regarding the child's skills and deficiencies. Some of these devices of assessment, which will be discussed in the course of the book include the following:

Formal, standardized measures of intellectual functioning, language behaviors, and achievement. Language-impaired children may indicate higher achievement in formal individual test situations than they demonstrate in everyday situations, or they may function better in daily tasks than they do in test situations. They may show significantly low scores in one area in relation to other areas, or they may display variability in scores from one test situation to another.

Analysis of the use, content, and form of expressive and receptive language. Spontaneous and elicited spoken and written samples should be used for analyzing each component of language and for studying integration of the components. Analysis should include observations within social interactions, formalized assessment procedures, and observations of written as well as spoken communication

Observations of the child in communication with other children. This provides different information about the child's communication behaviors than formal communication with the examining clinician provides.

Reports about the child regarding classwork, history, and use of free time. These can be obtained from the child, from the parents, and from the teacher for varying views of the child's weak and strong areas.

In some instances evaluation sessions do not give the clinician sufficient information for complete descriptions and understanding of the deficiencies. Occasionally it is useful to admit the child to a short trial period of intervention, which can include small-group work, classroom observation, informal conversation, and independent work assignments. In these situations behaviors may emerge that did not show up in the formal individual evaluation periods. Procedures and content of evaluation must be adapted to each individual (Miller, 1981), and it is extremely rare for one strategy or technique to provide comprehensive information regarding a child's language behaviors.

Discussion of evaluation usually implies an underlying assumption that a problem *does* exist. This is not always the case, of course. Some children *are* simply immature; some *are* uninterested in working merely because they are lazy or not motivated; some *are* slow in all areas without specific deficiencies in any areas; and, some parents *are* unnecessarily concerned. However, the subtleties of certain language disorders and the complexities of communication suggest that casual assessment is not in the best interest of any person suspected of having communication deficiencies. In the following section examples of specific procedures for qualitative analysis and standardized measures of quantitative evaluation are cited.

categorizing language deficiencies

The language components of use, content, and form will be considered throughout this discussion. The interrelatedness of language components in language acquisition and use makes it difficult to find categories for the various aspects of language and related behaviors. The type and severity of communication disorders are multi-faceted and defy unitary description. However, because of the complexities of language and language deviations, any discussion of the language system and communicative interactions requires agreement about terminology. For each component, language deviations are characterized in terms of deficiencies of *expression, reception,* and *organization.* Language-impaired children often exhibit characteristics that are too varied to describe as solely expressive, receptive, or organizational; for that reason, there is a fourth category labeled *combinatorial* deficiencies. Table 2–1 summarizes categories of language deviations useful for reference to either spoken or written communication.

Expressive Deficiencies These deficiencies involve inadequate spoken or written production of the intended message as judged by the linguistic and interactive rules of the context and situation. Expressive

TABLE 2–1

Categories of Language Deviations

EXPRESSIVE DEFICIENCIES	RECEPTIVE DEFICIENCIES	ORGANI- ZATIONAL DEFICIENCIES	COMBINA- TORIAL DEFICIENCIES
Inadequate production (spoken or written) of the intended message, as judged by linquistic and interactive rules of the context and the situation	Inadequate recognition of input (spoken or written) in terms of attaching significance, interpretation of sounds/letters, words and word combinations, and the relationships expressed in language	Inadequate planning or executing of goal-directed tasks	Any combination of inadequacies in the language system or its use for interpersonal or intrapersonal service

deviations are discussed in terms of *use, content,* and *form* as they appear in the speaker's native language (Bloom and Lahey, 1978; Nelson, 1981).

Use

Language use is the "reason for being" of language. All other aspects of language, including content and form, are selectively applied to utterances in order to use language efficiently and accurately. Language use includes:

1. Conveying the intent of the message through appropriate verbal and nonverbal devices for communicative interaction (that is, by selecting content, form, and gestures that fit the context and the situation)
2. Developing language competencies for intrapersonal growth, creativity, and direction and organization of behavior

Children with inadequate language use often do not integrate context and form to convey the intended messages in their interpersonal interactions, nor do they always observe the rules and customs of conversation. Each person's unique application of language within the social context of communication reflects interactive *style.* Normal speakers use language interactively in a way that is distinctly personal but is within the range of social and cultural acceptability. Language-impaired persons may perceive and convey experiences in mildly distorted ways that apparently reflect their communication inadequacies. Their manner of interacting with the world is distinguishable from non–language-impaired speakers and may represent stylistic distortions. The distinctive style which is observed in some language-impaired people may result from their inability to recognize appropriate ways to respond to or to express messages that the word meaning alone does not convey. The result of this inadequacy is often behavior that seems rude, uncaring, defiant, or just odd.

Content

Inadequate expression of *content* includes such inappropriate or inadequate use of words and word combinations that the compositional aspects of the message (combined meaning of words) and/or referential aspects of the message (word meaning) are not expressed appropriately.

Form

Expressive deficiencies of *form* include problems with the linguistic structures of spoken or written utterances, such as sound or letter formation, grammatical form, sentence types, and sentence complexity. Table 2–2 summarizes the categories of expressive-language deviations.

Receptive Deficiencies This term refers to inadequate recognition of spoken or written language input including attaching significance to the input, interpreting grammatical constructions, recognizing sounds or letters, understanding word meanings, and understanding relationships expressed in language. Receptive deficiencies are considered in terms of *use, content,* and *form* of the recipient's native language.

Use

Inadequate reception affecting use denotes misunderstanding or misinterpretation of the intent or function of a message sent by another person and may include the following:

1. Misinterpreting hidden or subtle messages
2. Misinterpreting indirect forms of request or instruction
3. Misunderstanding figurative uses of language and their relationship to the context of the message
4. Misreading speaker's signals, verbal and nonverbal that contribute to the message

TABLE 2–2

Categories of Expressive Language Deviations

DEFICIENCIES OF USE	DEFICIENCIES OF CONTENT	DEFICIENCIES OF FORM
Inadequate integration of language content and form for conveying the intent of the message and for intrapersonal development	Inadequate or inappropriate choice of words or word combinations to convey compositional meaning, and/or referential meaning	Inadequate expression of some or all aspects of linguistic structure, including sound or letter formation, grammatical constructions, sentence types, and sentence complexity

Content

Receptive deficiencies of content include:

1. Inadequate or incomplete understanding of word meanings (for example, misunderstanding referential meanings of words)
2. Inadequate understanding of compositional or propositional meanings (for example, relational meanings beyond word meanings)

Form

Receptive deficiencies of form include:

1. Inadequate recognition of sound or letter formations or combinations
2. Inadequate interpretation of grammatical constructions and their effect on meaning
3. Difficulty understanding differences in sentence types and their effect on meaning
4. Inadequate understanding of differences in sentence complexities and the compression of meaning into various sentence forms

Misinterpretation of form leads to misunderstanding of the meaning. Table 2–3 summarizes receptive deficiencies.

Organizational Deficiencies Inability to plan and/or execute tasks or a series of tasks directed toward a predetermined goal constitutes an organizational deficiency. Such a difficulty may occur even though the child understands and accepts the end goal. Discussions of organizational deficiencies are included in the sections on noncommunicative use of language.

Combinatorial Deficiencies Any combination of inadequacies in the language system or its use for interaction or personal development can be called a combinatorial deficiency.

The language deficiencies represented by these categories will be discussed in terms of some of their various characteristics, with implications for identification and assessment.

TABLE 2–3
Categories of Receptive Language Deviations

DEFICIENCIES OF USE	DEFICIENCIES OF CONTENT	DEFICIENCIES OF FORM
Inadequate interpretation of the intent or function of the message, spoken or written. The misunderstanding may involve misinterpretation of hidden or subtle messages or misreading speaker signals of movement, space, and phrasing	Inadequate or incomplete understanding of word meanings or the combinatorial propositions of words within the spoken or written context	Misinterpretation or inadequate recognition of phonological, grammatical or syntactical structures of language

expressive deficiencies: description and assessment

Some children with language-learning deficits understand what they hear but do not know how to say what they want to communicate. Children with expressive language dysfunction may not talk at all. They may speak telegraphically, using only high-content words; they may misarticulate sounds, missequence syllables or words in a sentence, or have difficulty relating an event they have experienced. Some language-impaired children are quite verbal but communicate ineffectively; others are excessively quiet. Many older language-impaired children answer questions and speak in well-structured utterances but do not know how to communicate the intent of their message to their listeners nor how to provide their listeners with necessary background information for the message.

Expressive Deficiencies of Use Except for some subtle qualities of language learning, children have acquired essentially adult knowledge of language by the time they are four or five (Bloom, 1974). From preschool age to about ten years, they continue to refine their perception of cues in communication and to develop strategies for producing the best message for the situation (Muma, 1978). An important difference between the expressive language of the preschool child and the older child is in its use. The use of language can be dichotomized into the communicative and the non-communicative components. People participate in a variety of social interactions and incorporate language into those interactions (Simon, 1979).

Communicative uses of language can be discussed in terms of functions of language, direct and indirect speech acts, and conversational proficiency.

Functions of Language

Halliday (1977) categorized early use of child language (before three years of age) into three phases with their characteristic functions:

Phase I (before eighteen months)

Instrumental— language used to satisfy needs or get things done ("I wanna . . ."; "Gimme")

Regulatory— language used to exert control over the behavior of others ("Do that"; "Sit here")

Interactional— language used to interact with others or in attempts to get along with others ("Hello"; "You and me")

Heuristic— language used to explore or understand the environment or learn new information ("What's that?"; "Why?")

Personal— language used to express self-identity, declare individuality, or express personal feelings ("Here I am"; "I don't like it")

Imaginative— language used to create imaginary or fantasy situations ("Let's play like")

Even though the child may not be combining words, or sometimes not even using words, the combination of vocalization, intonation, context, and nonverbal actions can be used to interpret the child's intentions. Halliday indicates that basic language functions are coordinated in later language development for more sophisticated function in dialogue:

Phase II (by two years)

Pragmatic— language used to act on reality (the language of doing), representing a combined use of instrumental, regulatory, and interactional function ("You get it")

Mathetic— language used to learn about the world or reflect on it (the language of learning), representing a combined use of personal, interactional, and heuristic functions ("It goes round like my record")

Informative— language used to convey content, making reference to objects or events in the world around the child ("That's a dog"; "I'll tell you")

Halliday suggests that by the time children are two years old they are engaging in dialogue by combining the elementary Phase I language functions to produce Phase II functions that are pragmatic, mathetic, or informative. His third phase identifies utterances that may be multi-functional:

Phase III (by three years)

Interpersonal— language used to relate with another person or discuss relationships ("We can get it")

Textual— language used to relate the form and content of preceding and following utterances ("You forgot to read that part")

Ideational and experiential— language used to convey thoughts or experiences to a listener ("My dad gave me a ball")

Miller (1981, p. 120) summarizes Halliday's description of language function in the following way:

"Halliday's view of language function . . . entails: (1) a developmental sequence in the emergence of the . . . basic functions; (2) reorganizations of the relations between form and function during development; and (3) multiple functions associated with multiword utterances." In normal school-age children and adults, linguistic acts usually serve more than one function simultaneously (Halliday, 1977; Chapman, 1978). For example, the utterance "I aced out on that test again" serves multiple functions, including the message (I scored well); acknowledgement of shared information about the past (*that* test); word meanings common to the communicators ("aced"); and implied happiness about the message.

Language-deficient children do not always exhibit well-developed language functions and may be limited to primitive language functions: ("here me," personal; "momma, stop it," regulatory; "you live here?", heuristic). The functional simplicity of utterances of language-impaired children often is apparent. Coordination of basic functions and the structural organization for conveying those functions is required for more sophisticated and effective communication than many language-deficient children demonstrate.

As Halliday (1977) suggests, young children learn they can represent ideas or objects with words. As they discover the separation of the symbol from the actual idea or object, they learn the content and form for conveying meanings and intentions. Children learn that movements and utterances affect people and influence their interaction with others; they learn how to structure their utterances to meet their communication needs. As normal-speaking children acquire more complex speech skills, they need more complex differentiation of communication acts (Miller, 1981). They no longer express events and objects in the present but begin to convey meanings and intentions not related to the current and the visible.

Communication and Speech Acts.

Communication acts include expressing thoughts or needs, asking questions, acting on the environment to change it, initiating contact with others, etc. (Halliday, 1977; Dore, 1974; Rees, 1978; Miller, 1981). Searle (1976) describes speech acts as the basic units of communication, including components of comprehension, expression, and utterance intentions. His descriptions of these units includes:

1. *Utterance acts (uttering words or sentences).* This unit apparently represents the syntactical or morphological components.
2. *Propositional acts (referring and predicting).* This unit seems to designate the semantic or content components.
3. *Illocutionary acts (commanding, promising, stating, questioning, and so on).* This unit represents use of language in which a speaker expects the listener to interpret the message (Rees, 1978; Simon, 1979).
4. *Perlocutionary force (being persuaded, convinced, alarmed).* This unit represents the effects utterances have on the hearer's actions, thoughts, or beliefs (this will be discussed in the section on receptive use of language).

An important way to consider expressive-language use is through analysis of the speaker's communicative intents—the reasons *why* people talk (illocutionary force). English verbs specifying illocutionary acts include "state," "assert," "warn," "remark," "command," "request," "criticize," "apologize," "demand," "argue," and so forth. Austin (1962), an originator of the idea of illocutionary acts, indicates that the English language contains more than a thousand expressions that can perform illocutionary acts. Dore (1977) describes several communicative intentions, or illocutionary acts, identifiable in early child communications:

1. Requests—asking for information or actions ("What's that?")
2. Responses—related to previous utterances ("His name's Zeke")
3. Descriptions—characterizing features of the information ("A red one")
4. Statements—expressing facts, emotions, and so on ("I like it")
5. Conversational devices regulating contact—controlling aspects of the interaction ("Now you do it")
6. Performatives—accomplishing acts by saying them ("You can't do it")

Rees (1978, p. 200) provides examples of some of the numerous other identifiable illocutionary acts:

Utterance	Illocutionary Act
This chowder is delicious.	Evaluating
Please take out the garbage.	Requesting
You were right about the mosquitoes.	Admitting

As these examples illustrate, speakers expect their utterances to be interpreted in a certain way; that is, they express something with the intention that the utterance will function in a particular way in the interaction. If a speaker asks a question, he or she may expect it to be answered, result in an action, or have some other effect, depending on the illocutionary force. If a speaker expresses a belief, he or she may expect the listener to understand that it is true, or he or she may intend to convince the listener, defend a position, or influence the listener's opinion. An important aspect of learning to communicate is learning to combine the content of the message with its intended impact. As they become proficient communicators, English language speakers learn to convey intent through both *direct* and *indirect* speech acts.

Conversational Proficiency

Communicative competence includes conversational proficiency, which requires the integration of linguistic skills with nonverbal information, prior context, and social situation (Rom and Bliss, 1981). Conversation must be a cooperative venture or communication will probably break down. Speakers and listeners make assumptions regarding what others know and expect from conversational interaction. Grice (1975) described categories of expectations, or rules, for the conversational event:

1. quantity of information to be provided
   a. provide enough information for the listener's needs
   b. do not give excessive information to the listener

2. quality of truthfulness of information to be provided
   a. do not say what is not believed to be true
   b. do not provide unsubstantiated information (for example, do not represent opinion as fact)
3. relevance to the topic
4. understandable, clear messages
   a. avoid ambiguity
   b. avoid obscuring the message
   c. provide logical order to the message

Grice notes that if these expectations are not met (that is, if the conversational rules are violated) the listener attempts to determine the speaker's implied meaning. For example, if a speaker lies (violation of the second rule), he or she may intend to mislead the listener. However, as Dore, Gearhart, and Newman point out (1978, p. 353), conversational rules usually are exploited to "convey meaning to the listener that goes beyond the literal meaning of the proposition of the utterance." Grice's theory has been used to explain how speakers and listeners recognize and express humor through deliberate violations of aspects of language use, content, and form (Dore, Gearhart, and Newman, 1978). Horgan (1981) also describes the deliberate violation of aspects of language for the purpose of being humorous. She notes that children must recognize semantic categories (classes of objects such as animate/inanimate) and phonological, syllabic, syntactic, and morphological patterns, and be willing to alter those patterns purposefully in an attempt at humor. Children who are aware of conventional language patterns and multiple word meanings, and their importance in social context, may elect to interact by humorous violation of a conversational or linguistic rule

Visiting Relative	*Child Attempting Humor*
You ve *grown a foot* since I've seen you!	No, I still have *two*.

Parent	*Child Attempting Humor*
Get on your clothes.	OK. I'll *stand* on them.

Use of humor by normal-speaking children represents the purposeful violation of conversational and/or linguistic rules. This can be contrasted with the literal interpretation of the message by language-impaired children, who are restricted in their comprehension and use of words and language function.

The analysis of competent versus incompetent communication in conversation has led to the development of models for describing communication attempts. For example, Loban (1963) observed more than 300 kindergarten through sixth-grade children and described at least three factors of communication proficiency:

1. *Fluency*—ability to choose and readily express utterances, including range of vocabulary items, precision of word choice, variety of statements, application of appropriate grammatical structure for the message, and freedom from dysfluency (or "mazes") within utterances
2. *Coherence*—organization of content with appropriate sentence construction (complexity of utterance as demanded by the message), sequencing of the message, and general ease in formulating and expressing the message
3. *Effectiveness and control*—the degree of interaction of language structure, choice of content words, and delivery of the message for its efficient communication

Simon (1979) incorporates Loban's description of coherence in conversation into a device for evaluating a child's fluency. She defines Loban's use of mazes, or dysfluency, as the "confused or tangled use of words when attempting to express a message" (p. 55). Simon characterizes mazes in terms of hesitations, false starts, and useless repetitions. Her description of Loban's mazes is summarized as follows:

1. Short mazes at the initiation of utterances ("I'm gonna . . . I'm gonna . . . I'm . . . um . . . gonna go with you.")
2. Short mazes in the middle of an utterance and related to it ("I was swimming, and . . . and . . . and we . . . and . . . it was raining.")
3. Long mazes not directly related to the utterance, as if the child had begun to relate something too difficult to continue ("I was watching TV, and the detective had to uh, when he was, uh, hum, not anybody, uh, the murder, uh . . . never mind.")

It appears that various levels of linguistic and social skills are required for conversational competence. Dore, Gearhart, and Newman (1978) suggest that utterances qualifying as *conversational acts* consist of illocutionary properties (intent of the utterance), content (proposing word meaning or referencing acts or objects), and grammatical structures. They propose that a conversational sequence involves a series of conversational acts with a common topic, accomplishes interactive purposes, and meets mutual conversational needs. People who engage in dialogue enter into an "elaborate social contract," including how to take turns, when to change topics, how to provide the listener information necessary for the conversation, and how to repair communication breakdowns (Donahue, Pearl, and Bryan, 1980, p. 388). Speakers attempt to convey the message for the listener's benefit;

listeners try to relate background information and new information to interpret the message. Components of conversational interaction discussed in this section include:

1. Dialogue and turn taking
2. Topic maintenance in conversation
3. Providing the listener with the information necessary for the conversation (for instance, filling the requirements of presupposition)
4. Repairing communication breakdowns
5. Observing conventional ways of interacting, depending on the person, situation, and topic

DIALOGUE AND TURN TAKING. Face-to-face talk is a social encounter and therefore involves customs and rules of the linguistic community that must be observed. Taking a turn in conversation is an important rule of dialogue which involves more than waiting one's turn while another finishes. According to Dore, Gearhart, and Newman, the design of turn taking affects what is said, when something is said, and how participants interact when talking to one another. In other words, the speaker must "construct his turn such that it is related to surrounding turns" (Dore, Gearhart, and Newman, 1978, p. 359), and the utterances acknowledge previous content and manner of presentation. The principles of turn taking can be illustrated in the following ways:

Principles of Turn Taking	Examples
Influence on *what* is said	ensuring no overlap of content
	acknowledging previous utterance by taking turns. (I was going to say that, but she already did; so I'll only agree and elaborate.)
Influence on *when* something is said	collaborating on the topic
	honoring the system of turn taking by not taking the other's turn prematurely (I want to change the topic now, but he's acting like he's not finished with this topic. I won't interrupt until he's finished.)
Influence on *how* something is said	providing feedback for the conversational partner (She's not listening to me, so I'm going to repeat my point louder and more slowly.)

Sacks, Schegloff, and Jefferson (1974) suggest that turn taking influences topic maintenance because in conversation it provides: (1) motivation for listening—(if one must participate in a conversation, one must attend to prior utterances) and, (2) a vehicle for indicating one's understanding of the message.

TOPIC MAINTENANCE IN CONVERSATION. One of the most impor-
tant points in analyzing conversation is the appropriateness of the response
relative to the speaker's utterance (for example, the appropriate continua-
tion of a conversational topic) (Wiig and Semel, 1980). Blank and Franklin
discuss the appropriateness of an utterance in terms of speaker/listener
interaction. They note that in a dialogue the listener repeatedly takes the
role of speaker. However, having been the listener immediately prior to
becoming the speaker places limits on the subject and manner of response.
If the listener hears a question ("What is your favorite color?"), the responses are fairly limited, and it would be disconcerting to the speaker if the
listener responded without adhering to the constraints of the topic ("I like
crackers with peanut butter"). An absence of response would also be unset-
tling to the questioner. The ability of the listener to deal with constraints
of the speaker's utterances depends on knowledge of conversational appropriateness (for example, knowing when to maintain the topic) (Blank and
Franklin, 1980).

Many language-impaired children demonstrate difficulty with the turn-
taking responsibilities of cooperative games, team sports, and shared work
activities; they also have difficulty accommodating the turn taking and topic
maintenance processes of conversation. Language-deficient children frequently act as if they are engaging in a monologue and do not respond to
—or elicit—comments from their conversational partners.

PRESUPPOSITIONS—PROVIDING INFORMATION FOR THE LISTENER.
The presupposition, or information that is assumed to be shared by speaker
and listener, is another important component of conversation. For successful communication to occur, the speaker and listener must share knowledge
and the speaker must gauge the listener's needs for specificity or background information (de Villiers and de Villiers, 1978; Greenfield and Zukow, 1978). Olson and Nickerson (1978, p. 118) suggest that ordinary
conversation only provides some cues to the speaker's intentions, because
what is said is only a "fragmentary representation of what is meant." They
discuss several aspects of presupposition that speakers and listeners must
consider in providing each other with enough information.

Aspects of presupposition include:

1. Shared knowledge, inclusive of prior knowledge, world knowledge, and
   listener-specific knowledge
2. Shared experiential context of the moment when the utterance is expressed
3. Preceding utterances in the conversation
4. Assumed listener biases
5. Numerous nonverbal clues regarding the speaker's intentions

It seems difficult for some language-impaired people to provide their listeners with a frame of reference for a conversation; consequently they often are described as vague, out-to-lunch, or someone who makes you feel that you've entered the conversation in the middle. The language-deficient person may not know what the listener knows and needs to know, nor how to fill that communication gap between oneself and the listener. Language-impaired children may have difficulty providing the most informative elements of the message; they may give misleading or partial information, or fail to convey adequate references to objects, events, or people. When language-impaired children do not fill the requirements of presupposition, they often leave their listeners baffled: "He went there and hit him," the child mentions at breakfast. The listener may not know who "he" is, where "he" went, or if the hitting happened at school, in a dream, or last year.

The understanding of shared speaker/listener elements includes aspects of time and place, as well as references to persons and objects. Language-impaired children sometimes fail to provide those references, acting as if the listener has shared all their cognitive and literal experiences. In some instances the language-impaired child omits semantic referents that are needed for the listener to understand the complete message, forcing the listener to question the child for necessary information. For example:

Adult	*Child*
	Tracy want to go to a Mexican.
What did you say? She wants what?	To go to a Mexican.
To a person?	No, to eat.
To a Mexican *place*?	Yes, to eat nachos and cheese on it.

Adult	*Child*
	If you burn it, you put it on.
Burn what?	Here. *(points to neck)*
How did you burn your neck?	In the sun. You put on your burn.
You put something on your burn?	Then it won't burn.
What do you put on it?	Lotion.

Adult	*Child*
What else did you buy besides a bow and arrow?	A Indian.
You bought an Indian?	*(nods)*
A person?	A hat.
You bought an Indian *hat*?	Yes, for my head.

Linguistic devices that signal speaker-specific information are also very important to conversation.

DEIXIS. This is a term denoting the linguistic forms that indicate locations relative to the speaker, the persons who are and are not participating in the conversation, and the time of occurrence relative to the conversation (Rees, 1978). Deixis, or the linguistic coding of the person, place, or time relative to the conversation, and speaker-specific information about location, can be illustrated in the following ways (de Villiers and de Villiers, 1978; Rees, 1978; Wiig and Semel, 1980):

Person	Place	Time	Space
personal	this	verb tense	near
pronouns	that		close
	here		
	bring		around
	take		behind

The appropriate use of deictic markers to provide the listener with adequate perspective for the conversation is learned only in conversation. Normal-speaking children engage in playlike and role-playing situations, which provide them with the framework for learning the use of deictic terms. Very young and language-impaired children sometimes fail to use deictic markers appropriately. "Is Mary *here*?" the language-impaired child asks the person who answers the telephone.

In the course of any conversation, interruptions and distractions can cause a breakdown in communication. When communication does break down (for instance, the listener responds inappropriately; the speaker forgets a word or key point) the conversational partners usually try to repair the conversation.

REPAIRING COMMUNICATION BREAKDOWNS—REVISION STRATEGIES. The strategy of revising an utterance to accommodate the listener's needs is important to conversational interaction. Each conversational partner is obligated to inform the other of failure to send or receive a message ("I didn't hear you." "*Who* said that?"). Partners must monitor the message, and given any interferences in the conversation's transmission or reception, attempt to:

Signal the disruption to the other ("*What* did you say?" "That's not what I said.")

Begin to repair the breakdown ("I didn't hear *whom* you said." "I *meant* that. . . .)

Normal speakers learn at an early age to meet conversational obligations by requesting clarification or restating an utterance. Garvey (1977) reported that children as young as preschool age request information from a speaker within conversational situations. Very young children (before preschool age) often do not request additional information from a speaker even though they may realize the inadequacy of the information received (Donahue, Pearl, and Bryan, 1980). Language-impaired children may not provide or request necessary clarifying information when needed. One study by Bryan and Pflaum (1978) required language-learning disabled children in fourth and fifth grades to teach games to a classmate and to a younger child. The language-learning impaired children did not modify instructions to accommodate their listeners' needs. When language-deficient children did recognize the ambiguity of messages (for example, they didn't understand the exact message), they did not clarify it (by repetition, rephrasing, and so on).

Language-impaired children exhibit several deficiencies in repairing communication breakdowns, including the following:

1. They are less able to consider the listener's perspective when producing the message (Donahue, Pearl, and Bryan, 1980). (Apparently related to the use of presuppositional aspects of conversation and of deictic markers)
2. They do not honor the conversational rules for monitoring and repairing communication breakdown (for example, signaling the occurrence of disrupted communication; "I didn't hear you."; or modifying the utterance for the listener, "I *said*. . . . ")

Many language-impaired children who attempt to engage in conversational acts display inadequate linguistic and/or social skills for successful participation in communicative interaction.

CONVENTIONS, CODES, AND STYLES—LANGUAGE USE AND SOCIAL BEHAVIOR. Language-impaired children often exhibit distinctive behaviors which experienced clinicians readily identify as characteristic of a person with language impairment. Deficiencies in the social behavior of language-disordered children are described in terms of their inadequacies in language functions, failure to observe turn-taking rules, lack of attempts to repair communication breakdowns, and ignoring the requirements of presuppositions. The problem may include difficulty interpreting the social environment, difficulty estimating space and territorial boundaries in interactions, and problems in responding to situations requiring specific behaviors (Wiig and Semel, 1976). Many language-deficient people stand too close, talk too loudly, and divulge family secrets unexpectedly. These and other social misbehaviors appear in language-deficient people of all ages. Kalgill, Friedland, and Shapiro (1973) observed that good predictors of learning disorders in kindergarten children were immaturity, poor social and emotional adjustment, and impulsive behavior, as well as problems with speech and language. Apparently the casual observer's judgments of behaviors often take the form of social symptoms or labels (immature); however, the language specialist should not be misled or jump to conclusions about emotional development until all facets of language have been assessed.

Social and interpersonal problems increase for language-impaired children when they reach puberty. Physical changes require changes in behavior; other people's expectations of them change. The language-impaired adolescent may be unaware of the nonverbal aspects of interaction, particularly those with potential sexual connotations. The young person may send out unintended messages or receive information that is not interpreted as intended. For example, a language-impaired adolescent may stare at someone, or hold eye contact for a long time in an attempt to gain information about a person. The directness and length of the gaze may embarrass the recipient or be interpreted as an invitation for more intimate interaction. Innocent movements and gestures, such as absentmindedly touching one's own body parts while talking, or touching another person, may be misinterpreted by a listener and create some startling situations for the language-impaired adolescent.

The language user must know the rules for language application within the social context as determined by variables of social situation, conversational topic, sex, rank, age, social class, and familiarity (Berko Gleason, and Weintraub, 1978).

The use of *codes* in interactions involves the modification of utterances by a speaker for conveying the desired effect of a message in a certain situation. Speakers must exercise options about the ways in which they will produce their messages. Learning to select the appropriate code for the context and the listener is an important aspect of interaction. We observe children's utterances, often described as "frank" or "honest," that display an inappropriate choice of code for the message and the listener.

> "You're too fat to sit in that little chair" *(spoken to an aunt)*
>
> "I hope I never get as old as you are!" *(spoken to a grandmother)*

Statements like these represent failure to choose alternate codes more approrpiate to the circumstances:

> "This chair will be more comfortable"
>
> "I don't want to get older"

People within linguistic and social communities understand the rules governing the application of codes. Normal speakers and listeners elect to alter the way in which the message is delivered, changing from one code to another depending on the listener and the situation.

> "Gimme some money" *(spoken to a brother)*
>
> "May I borrow a dollar until tomorrow?" *(spoken to a father)*

Joos (1976) describes five codes (which he terms "styles," but which are consistent with the use of the term "code" in this discussion), summarized as follows:

1. *Frozen*— apparently this is the most distant, noninteractive form of communicative code, and may represent language exchanges that never vary (ritualistic recitations)
2. *Formal*— designed to inform with no participation from the listener (introductions, lectures)
3. *Consultative*— used with strangers; speaker supplies background information (response to an information-seeking question)
4. *Casual*— used with acquaintances and friends in conversation; minimal background information in the context
5. *Intimate*— excludes public information (a "family joke"); each intimate group invents its own code

Joos notes that a speaker is free to shift from one code to another even within one utterance; however, only two neighboring codes can be used sequentially. It appears antisocial to shift two or more steps within a single utterance. For example, a speaker shifting two steps from formal to casual presentation might shock his/her listener by changing the emphasis from what is said to how it is said, obscuring the intended message. "Mr. Smith, I need to discuss the teacher's job descriptions and salaries with you." (formal) "Do you dig me, Joe?" (casual).

In certain situations, a code shift is used as a humorous or poetic device, but it is neither humorous nor poetic when a child or adolescent does not understand the basic use of codes and executes changes that disrupt communicative contact and interfere with the intended message. Interpersonal relationships are important determinants of conversational code choice. Different interpersonal relationships require different choices (Fielding and Fraser, 1978). Some language-deficient people fail to observe the conventional formulas appropriate for their message, situation, and listener.

> A young language-impaired woman was describing to her clinician her emotional pain regarding a particular family problem. The two were involved in an intense interaction when the language-impaired woman said, as part of the discussion about Tom, "Tom . . . he's my brother . . . was at my house when it happened."

Of course, Tom's identity was shared information and had been part of the clinician's knowledge for years (see discussion regarding presupposition). The sudden reminder of this information was inappropriate and represented a noticeable shift in communicative code (from intimate to formal and back to intimate).

Often, language-impaired children exhibit a limited range of communicative interactions; their behavior may be stereotypic and idiosyncratic, and they may speak without changing pitch or tone (Wiig and Semel, 1980).

The ability to modify one's speech according to the listener is acquired relatively early (Schatz and Gellman, 1973; Sacks and Devin, 1976). Children as young as four years old make changes in their speech to babies that are roughly parallel to the changes adults make in their speech to young children. The sentences are shorter, key words are more heavily emphasized, and attention-getting devices are used more often (Sacks and Devin, 1976). Modifications in speech form and word choice made on the basis of the listener's age and linguistic ability are common to adult speakers (Fey, Leonard, and Wilcox, 1981).

Using *indirect speech acts* is a way of manipulating utterances to affect interactions. As the young child's speech develops, vocabulary expands and the structure accommodates increasing complexities of meaning and intentions. The child's awareness of the listener's knowledge also expands. From this awareness comes the child's understanding of the effect utterances can have on the listener, and how the manipulation of those utterances affects personal interaction. In this sense, the function of an utterance is distinguished from the propositional content (de Villiers and de Villiers, 1978). For example, comments that appear superficially to be a request for information ("Can you shut the door?") are not intended to request, but to convey a polite version of a command. The utterance, then, means something other than what it says. Often in English the direct purpose of the utterance is disguised by phrases formulated for politeness. In some way, very young children express and interpret the propositional aspects of utterances instead of the intended version (Ervin-Tripp, 1977). Language-impaired children often do not use or interpret the intent of an utterance.

Clinician	Language Impaired Child
"Don't spill the beans."	"OK. I'm a good cook."

A difficult lesson for some language-deficient children to learn is that utterances do not always mean what they say, and that the content of an utterance alone does not provide the necessary cues for its interpretation.

Prekindergarten language learners acquire facility with idioms and figurative uses of speech, but many language-deficient children fail to use or interpret anything but the most literal meanings of words.

Interactive style represents each speaker's combination of language use, content, and form, as displayed within the boundaries of cultural and social appropriateness. Style is the result of interaction between verbal and non-verbal aspects of communication within the framework of the context and situation. For example, the way a speaker chooses and combines words for the exact purpose of the message, attends to the listener, uses his/her body and voice as part of the interaction—all contribute to the communicator's individual style. When language serves as a tool in the dynamics of human interaction, the communicative process is affected by the adequacy of the language system. If the language system is impaired, then the communication the language is serving may be distorted. If a child does not know how to adjust the communication code for the listener or situation, does not participate in turn-taking protocol, does not provide the listener with enough information, or does not try to repair interrupted communication, then the interaction is affected. Language-deficient people often fail in some or all of these conversational skills, and their lack of awareness represents a distinctive style.

Traditionally, assessment and intervention programs have neglected the child's interpersonal application of language. Language-deficient children must learn to attend not only to what they say and how they say it, but how they look and sound while saying it. In clinical situations, we see language-impaired children grow into adolescents and adults who do not develop an awareness of other people's feelings, and who do not acquire ways of expressing their own emotions. The personalities of language-impaired people appear bizarre sometimes, especially in communicative interaction.

Words serve in combination with other tools of communication, including nonverbal skills, previous information, unspoken messages, and contextual and situational features of the interaction (*Asha,* 1980). Some of the expressive, nonverbal characteristics influencing the communication act include:

1. Getting the other person's attention
2. Providing nonverbal clues to the message or intent (intonation, gestures, pausing, rate variation, pitch change)
3. Speaking with appropriate loudness while looking at the listener

The slightest gesture (rolling one's eyes, shrugging one's shoulders) can help the listener interpret a message, particularly in the event of conflicting verbal messages: "I guess he doesn't know the answer" (spoken by the teacher with a wink and a grin while pointing to a child who is wildly waving his hand).

Normal speakers use a combination of verbal and nonverbal signals to convey their messages; they learn this ability before they reach preschool.

For example, Jones (1975) describes a wide repertoire of facial expressions and gestures of nursery school children who apparently display highly complex nonverbal interaction. Jones discusses differences between talking, shouting, and singing, as well as other noises accompanying communication in children. Language-impaired people do not always observe or use nonlinguistic information that affects the verbal message, such as pitch change, stress on certain words, facial expressions, or rate change.

Normal speakers interpret behaviors as part of the message; many messages sent and/or received by language-impaired children set off distorted, bizarre, and even comical interchanges. The child may misuse a word or misinterpret an utterance in the classroom. The teacher then reads the misinterpretation as deliberate, particularly if the child's reaction is stated in quick, blunt terms with a shoulder shrug. This breach of classroom conduct by what seems to be an insolent child creates a reaction in the teacher who then sends a message to the student: "You'd better look out." The child doesn't know exactly *how* to look out for *what*. He or she becomes irritated or anxious at the teacher's constant grumpy manner. The teacher in turn has identified a chronic smart aleck who doesn't exert any effort to be a "good" student.

In communicative interactions, style represents a blending of culture-appropriate behavior with the language system as it is used in communication. The rules of conversation include regard for physical distance and space during interaction, monitoring of the use of volume in speaking, and incorporation of nonverbal actions into the interchange. Language-deficient children may not note that different listener/speaker interactions require different codes and styles. When this happens, Listener A (the child's grandmother) may be given a message in the same way as Listener B (a younger brother). Language-deficient children frequently are considered rude, uncaring, or demanding when they merely lack a socially redeeming communication style. They fail to observe linguistic and nonlinguistic maxims of their linguistic community for appropriate interaction.

Some language-deficient children need direct teaching of both verbal and nonverbal social behaviors, particularly as expressed through the medium of language. Assessment should include notice of the language-deficient child's interactive styles. Speakers choose content and form of language partially on the basis of what is socially appropriate; language-impaired persons may not be able to interpret the situation well enough to know how to be appropriate.

Metalinguistic Skills

A crucial part of oral or written communication involves the ability to use language to analyze language. The process of appreciating and reflecting on language is referred to as *metalinguistic* behavior (de Villiers and de Villiers, 1978). As a child approaches school age, he/she displays aware-

ness of language as a system to be studied and used; metalinguistic awareness is acquired long after the child demonstrates the application of
adequate linguistic behaviors (de Villiers and de Villiers, 1978). Metalinguistic skills include awareness of component sounds, syllables, and words;
awareness of grammatical and semantic rules; recognition of the interactive
use of language; and the use of language for learning.

When the normal-speaking child reaches five or six years of age, communication skills are sophisticated, and he/she has become aware of language
as a tool to be manipulated and talked about. Five-year-old children learn,
for example, that language can be played with (to make up words and *talk
about* making up *words;* to play rhyming games and *talk about* how funny it
sounds; used to lie or pretend (knowing they didn't "*say*" the truth); used
to ask about the words on paper ("What does it *say?*")

Metalinguistic awareness of sounds, words, or word combinations includes conscious recognition that words are composed of component parts.
Even though listening and speaking skills have developed on the basis of
those components, recognition is not conscious until a child is about five
years old (de Villiers and de Villiers, 1978). The de Villiers note that until
a child is able to separate words from things, reading and writing present
problems. The child must be able to conceive of a word as a *word,* or a
symbol removed from the actual object, and be able to refer to the word or
utterance itself. Until this occurs the child has difficulty treating the written
word as an equivalent referent to the spoken word. Formal schooling usually
begins about the time most children acquire the necessary metalinguistic
awareness for transferring oral language to written form. Beilin (1975)
notes that reading requires the child to shift attention from one aspect of
the word to another (from word meaning to sound components to letter
equivalents). Other academic subjects also require metalinguistic skills; the
child often must transfer the spoken or written language symbol to another
symbol system such as chemical, mathematical, or musical.

Frequently language-deficient children are not aware of language as separate from context, or as a system that can be talked about and analyzed.
Therefore, talking to them about what they didn't "say" correctly has little
impact. They may have difficulty segmenting sounds from words when they
hear the combined sounds and are asked what "word" they make. They may
not be able to make up words, create rhymes, correct errors in things they
say, make a linguistic mistake on purpose, or play games with words (*Asha,*
1980). Metalinguistic tasks, for example, require the person to remove
himself/herself from the usual meaning of a word ("dog") and attend to the
properties of the words ("what *sounds like* dog?") (Blank, 1978). Metalin-
quistic tasks may require one to shift focus to alternative uses, alternative
meanings, or to the grammatical construction. Metalinguistic abilities of
using utterances beyond their singular, referential meaning—as required
for games, humor, correcting errors, or judging ambiguities—are important

for academic progress and social interaction. Language-impaired children must be frequently instructed in the nature of metalinguistic tasks which requires metalinguistic awareness before correction will have much effect ("You didn't *say* that word right." "What *sound* does that *word* start with?").

Summary of Expressive Language Use In Interaction

In the first four or five years of life, a child's language evolves into a flexible tool for interaction and learning. In the preschool years the child is able to:

1. Modify the content of utterances for the listener's benefit
2. Converse about events out of the immediate situation
3. Alter communication codes for different listeners

Demands increase for the child to apply language to more varied and more complex interactions and learning situations. The normal-speaking five year old or six year old becomes aware of sounds and words as components of communication and can manipulate language for play and learning. Assessment of language use should take these factors into account.

Assessment of Expressive Language Use: Quantitative Methods

Standardized measures of language use that provide normative data for statistical analysis are rare. A few criterion-referenced measures are available that compare the child's semantic and pragmatic skills with normal sociolinguistic development. *The Behavioral Inventory of Speech Act Performance* (Lucas, 1977) was designed to assess a child's use of the form and meaning of language.

Assessment of Expressive Language Use: Qualitative Methods

The communicative acts that language serve may be independent of the literal meaning and syntactic constructions of the utterances. Determining the effectiveness of a child's use of language in communication must include qualitative analysis of the child's verbal and nonverbal behaviors during the performance of speech acts and an evaluation of effectiveness in conveying the intended message. The situation, context, interpersonal interactions, and time of observations should be varied to provide adequate information for assessment (Wiig and Semel, 1980; Miller, 1981). Assessment of communicative competence involves the consideration of communication intentions (for example, requesting information, clarifying) as well as conversational effectiveness. Lucas (1980 pp. 86–87) provides a set of questions for the clinician to consider in determining a child's expressive semantic and pragmatic abilities. Questions that seem to pertain to the pragmatic use of language are summarized as follows:

1. Does the child use a variety of lexical items to express various communicative functions? (for example, choice of appropriate words for the intent of the message)?
2. Are the child's utterances appropriate for the situation and context?
3. Does the child express a variety of speech acts, such as requesting, denying, asserting, stating information?

Current literature in the assessment of communicative effectiveness emphasizes the gathering of spontaneous and "free speech" samples for analysis (Simon, 1979; Lucas, 1980; Miller, 1981). Miller (1981) details the processes of collecting and recording reliable speech samples. He includes obtaining a representative record of the child's usual productive language, the nature of the interaction recorded, the setting, the materials for enhancing free speech, the methods of accurately recording what the child produces, and examples of sample size and context. Simon (1979) also discusses examples of language sample notations and offers illustrations of incompetent communication. Examples that seem to pertain to language use are summarized as follows:

1. Use of restricted versus elaborated code (after Bernstein, 1972) that involves situational-bound communication rather than content free of immediate context, such as departure into an imaginary story
2. Coherence of ideas so that main thoughts are clear and subordinate points are organized as parts of main ideas
3. Establishment of a story line from imagination and pursuit of the theme
4. Interaction of information with appropriate structure and word choice to fulfill the intent of the message
5. Fluency of expression with minimal interference from mazes and other fillers that do not contribute to the message
6. Maintenance of a dialogue, so that the child participates in the conversation by following the topic, clarifying a point for the listener, and checking the accuracy of information provided to the listener

The following represents a summary of Lucas's (1980) descriptions of ineffective communication skills as they relate to language use:

1. The child does not initiate verbalization to express needs (he/she may wait to be given toys, snacks, and other things rather then asking for them).

2. The child gives listener-inappropriate or misleading paralinguistic cues (for example, inappropriate stress for the message, inappropriate intensity of utterance, unrelated gestures, or prolonged insufficient eye contact).
3. The child usually does not specify referents, offering nonspecific or unreferenced utterances which the listener confused about the message or its intent.
4. The child uses physical means to solve problems when a few words would serve better (as examples, he/she becomes physically aggressive or excessively passive to change the situation or leaves the room or cries without expressing a reason for the needed change).

The uses of language for (inter)acting and for learning develop to complex levels in normal communicators, but in language-deficient children and adolescents either or both uses may be limited. Assessment of both oral and written language use should provide valuable information for intervention.

Noncommunicative Uses Of Language

Several important uses of language do not contribute directly to interpersonal interactions. Noncommunicative uses of language include information gathering, concept formation, questioning to test perceptions and hypotheses, self-direction, problem solving, and creating novel meanings (Rees, 1978). Halliday (1978) discusses the potential of language for extending one's resources to new situations. He suggest that creativity through language is not the construction of new sentences but is the use of language for the abstraction of experiences and the development of concepts. Many language impaired children do not develop their creativity through verbal channels, although verbal creativity may not be an impossibility for them.

Tough (1977) identified several major functions of language in preschool and school-age children that seem primarily related to the roles language plays in behavior, control, imaginative activities, and problem solving. Tough's functions, which are identified as directive, interpretive, projective, and relational, are summarized as follows:

Function	Uses	Strategies
Directive	self-directing	monitoring actions
		focusing control
		planning ahead
	other-directing	demonstrating actions requested
		instructing
		planning ahead
		anticipating collaborative action between self and another

Interpretative	reporting on current and past experiences	labeling
		elaborating detail
		associating and comparing with earlier detail
		recognizing incongruity
		being aware of sequence
	reasoning	recognizing causal relationships
		recognizing conditions for relationships
Projective	predicting	forecasting events
		anticipating consequences
		considering alternatives of action
		predicting related possibilities
		recognizing problems and predicting solutions
	empathizing	projecting into feelings or experiences of others
		anticipating the reactions of others
	imagining	renaming
		commenting on the imagined content
		fantasizing through language
		role playing through language
Relational	self-maintaining	expressing need
		projecting self-interest
		justifying actions
	interacting	criticizing
		threatening
		employing strategies emphasizing self or others

The language-impaired child often does not direct himself well although he may be very good at telling other people how to conduct their own lives. The ability to use language to consider one's thoughts and to organize one's behavior represents an intrapersonal use of language (Berko Gleason and Weintraub, 1978).

ORGANIZATION AND EXECUTION OF TASKS. Poor organization and execution of tasks are related to Tough's directive functions of language. Some language-impaired children have extreme difficulty monitoring their own actions, focusing their attention, planning ahead, and executing well-ordered actions. Getting through a regular day of school and chores is more difficult for the child who has poor skills in planning and executing tasks. Even though the language-impaired child may "spend hours" pursuing an activity of his/her own choosing, actions directed and designed by other people can pose real problems. As the child passes from kindergarten through the primary grades and into the middle grades, parents and teachers increasingly expect the child to take more independent responsibility for planning and carrying out actions. Some of the actions include printing letters and numbers without supervision, dressing, eating a meal without prompting, getting home with homework assignments, and accomplishing routine chores at home. It seems that children with organizational/planning problems understand the final product that is desired but cannot execute the component steps without constant monitoring. At least two phases of the breakdown in planning and execution can be identified.

> *Initiating a task*—some children seem unable to begin a task and rarely exercise independent initiation of one. When the children are pushed into action through external means ("start your math homework or else") they work for a short time and then stop until they again have external direction,
>
> *Maintaining action on a task over time*—some children are self-starting but seem unable to maintain production until task completion. They write the first three words or work the first two math problems, then drift away from the task.

It seems that to some children executing a series of chores, or completing a long-term school project where the steps are not given one at a time, presents insurmountable obstacles. Grades suffer because assigned work is not completed; family interactions deteriorate because the child appears careless and irresponsible. Some children with this problem even need supervision in their free time to prevent aimless wandering. It is as though they had no internal signals about time or the passage of time as it relates to their activities. Their attention drifts, they sit for long periods without any observable action, and then they are really surprised when they are chastised for not completing their work.

Teachers and parents often find this type of problem frustrating and difficult to handle.

> One-to-one she's fine, but in a group or by herself she can't get anything done. She is a very honest and trustworthy child . . . except when it comes to school work. She has been very dishonest with me and her teachers about homework, test grades, etc.

He'd be passing all his subjects if he'd just get his assignments in. He doesn't finish anything. He gets high achievement test scores but daydreams his way through every class. He can only do timed tests. All attempts to help him do succeed—but only for a week.

I lay out his clothes at 7:00 every morning and tell him to get dressed. At 8:30 he isn't even finished putting on one sock.

She acts like she doesn't even know how to play. If she has a friend over to play who tells her what to do, she's fine, but if she's supposed to entertain herself, she wanders around asking me what to do.

Frequently, organizational deficits of the nature just described have companion features.

1. Difficulty executing/coordinating any two simultaneous activities (reaching for a book while erasing a mark)
2. Trouble integrating information from one sensory pathway to another (reaching for a book while trying to listen to a teacher's instructions)

It seems that organizing more than one thing at a time, or attending to more than one unit of information at a time, is too much for some children. Some children learn to perform each task consciously, "talking" themselves through the motions, as though nothing can be done automatically. The necessary actions can be performed with conscious self-direction and awareness of the tasks to be accomplished, but any distraction interrupts the effort.

The conscious planning of actions, as contrasted with the automatic way many people carry out actions or tasks, can be illustrated in the following way:

Imagine you suddenly found yourself driving across London. You are in the left lane of traffic with the steering wheel on the right side of the car. You could manage to drive across town without serious damage to yourself, but you would need to concentrate totally on your driving, and you probably would be tired at the end of the drive.

Ordinary driving in familiar circumstances requires little conscious effort from experienced drivers, who can drive miles without attending to the act of driving. They can listen to the radio, put on lipstick, comb their hair, or plan the day's work as they drive.

Most of us who are fairly well-integrated and organized perform hundreds of actions every day while thinking of something else. Children who have poor organization and movement planning skills seem unable to execute actions without conscious attention to each task. It is easy to imagine how other functioning suffers when one must attend focally to the execution of simple actions.

Disorganization problems are discussed by Lucas (1980) in terms of spatio-temporal difficulties in which children do not acquire the semantic skills for designating spatial and time dimensions. Lucas notes problems with such daily activities as following directions, completing assignments, explaining events, and learning new games. While many normal children seem to have an innate sense of the passage of time and an awareness of where their bodies are in relation to the rest of the world, many children with organizational deficits seem to have little semblance of an internal clock or an internal map of direction or sequence. Frequently, language analysis will show that the same disorganized children exhibit poor organization and presentation of both oral and written verbal material.

Expressive Deficiencies of Content Both oral and written language content include the meanings of individual words (referential components) and the meanings of word combinations (propositional aspects) (Halliday, 1973; Bates, 1976; de Villiers and de Villiers, 1978; Miller, 1981). Content can include the relationships between nouns and verbs in utterances and the appropriate word choices for the conveyance of meaning. Children must sort out which aspects of their experiences are relevant for a particular word or word combination in order to represent their worlds linguistically.

Words are *referential* when they refer to categories or subcategories of experience (animal, dog, collie) and an object can be referred to in many ways (pup, the cute mutt, the old hound). Adults and normal-speaking school-age children learn to choose the most appropriate word for the object and its referent (de Villiers and de Villiers, 1978). The propositional meanings of utterances (also called relational or compositional meanings) include intersentence relations, intrasentence relations, and contextual relations (Miller, 1981).

Referential Meanings of Words

Children must learn conventional linguistic symbols to represent different meanings (boy = young + male + human) and to observe restrictions on possible word combinations (one can say, for example, "the dog's paw," but not "the dog's wing," unless a joke is intended). They must also learn refinement to word meanings (big, dark-haired man).

Direct experience allows infants and young children to attain concepts that evolve into representation by verbal symbols (warm, soft, loud, sweet) (Carroll, 1980). In the course of a person's life, concepts become more complex as experiences expand the perceptual and cognitive boundaries of words. Children must learn to differentiate the various contexts in which a word can be used, recognizing differences in word meanings as well as in word combinations. Children learn words, or symbols, for objects, actions, and relationships among objects and their positions in space and time (de Villiers and de Villiers, 1978). Clark (1973) and McNeil (1970) discuss acquisition of word meaning in terms of semantic features. They describe consistencies in children's word usage and suggest that the addition of units of meaning (semantic features) to a word increases the complexity of a word (for example, the word "boy" encompasses the features *human* + *male* + *young* whereas the word "person" denotes only the feature *human*). The word "boy" therefore represents a more complex word because of the additional features. Brown (1973) and Bowerman (1978) also indicate that semantic complexity is a factor in word acquisition and affects order of acquisition among sets of semantically related words. Gentner (1975) notes that young children may interpret more complex words as if they were synonymous with less complex words, suggesting that they have not acquired the additional features needed to differentiate complexity. Language-impaired children often fail to make important distinctions in meaning represented by additional features of words that share some common features. For example, the verbs *pay* and *trade* are less complex semantically than the verbs *buy, sell,* and *spend,* which are acquired later on (Gentner, 1975). A young child, or a language-deficient child, might say, "I paid money for the coke, and I got it", whereas a more sophisticated speaker might say "I bought the coke."

Many language-deficient children acquire word meaning based on one property, such as a perceptual quality, and do not expand the word meaning to include properties of functionality (for example, what to do with it) or other subclasses of the broad category. Language-impaired children often do not learn the words for abstracting ideas, for representing their own feelings, or for representing experiences. Many language-deficient children acquire basic relationships (action, agent, object) but do not grasp more complex semantic relations or the linguistic forms for conveying the relations (Wiig and Semel, 1976; 1980). This often results in such expressive problems as misuse of words, problems finding words, limited usage of words and word combinations, adherence to concrete word and propositional meanings, and expression of only those references or propositions directly related to their own experiences of conditions. School-age children having difficulties with semantic relations usually exhibit difficulty not only with spoken and written expression, but also with tasks requiring expression of abstract relations, such as some of the quantitative relations used in mathematics (Lucas, 1980).

Words differ in the complexity of their application, as suggested by de Villiers and de Villiers (1978).

Proper names—representing only one referent for each word ("Mommy," "Dada," "Bobo")

Common names or nouns—applying to a class of objects with similarities (chairs, dogs)

Relational words—including dimensional attributes, such as "big," "tall," or "little." Correct application depends on a standard that varies with the object and the context. The child must identify the relevant properties of the object, as well as compare the object to the current standard (de Villiers and de Villiers, 1978)

Words indicating personal perspective (deictic expressions)—conveying to the listener the perspectives of time, position, and person as they relate to the speaker and the time an utterance is spoken. (As with other aspects of meaning, deixis is related closely to language use and is discussed in that section.)

In normal development of relationship terms and of categorical words that can be subcategorized, children begin with a global or categorical word (big) and gradually learn to refine and specify subcategories of the dimension (tall, long, fat). As they become adept in their use of dimensional terms, they use them in situations of differing relative standards. For example, a child learns that a sand box is *big* when asked to compare it to a match box, but *little* when asked to compare it to his/her own house. Language-deficient children sometimes learn to use global terms but do not refine or subcategorize their referents and do not shift standards when using words or expressing relative characteristics of objects. In the application of terms such as *big-little, long-short,* and *thick-thin,* very young speakers, as well as some language-impaired speakers, attend only to the global terms of size (for example, using *big* and *tall* synonymously). Dimensional terms such as *long* and *big* are learned early as global references, and the differentiations within classes of terms develop as language becomes more sophisticated *(long-short; tall-short)* (Donaldson and McGarrigle, 1974; Dore, 1974; Dale, 1976).

Propositional Meaning of Utterances

Conveying meaning requires the integration of individual word meaning with sentence and topic meaning to produce the composite meaning of the utterance. Compositional or propositional meaning takes into consideration the interactions among words, such as agents *(doers)*, actions, and objects of the actions. These word associations are termed semantic relations and represent meaning, or propositions, expressed through selected word combinations (Fillmore, 1968; Lucas, 1980). Miller (1981) divides relational meanings into three levels: intrasentence relations, intersentence relations, and contextual relations.

Intrasentence relations, as defined by Miller, involve the semantic roles of sentence constituents such as those represented by the following broad semantic categories:

Agent—initiator or actor

Location—place or position in space

Action—perceived movement

Object—recipient of action or force of activity

Possessor—owner of something

Attribute—characteristic or quality of something

These semantic categories, adapted from Fillmore (1968), Chafe (1970), Brown (1973), and Miller (1981), form the basis for early word combinations used to signal compositional meanings. Children use word combinations to express associations and attributes among people, objects, actions, or processes. More complex intrasentence relations are expressed by joining two propositions within one utterance, such as "She *came and got* the ball." The conjoining of propositions from one sentence to another occurs when children use compound and/or complex utterances (for example, two sentences made into one), such as "She lost the ball at home." + "She came home with the ball." = "She lost the ball after she got home."

Johnston and Kamhi (1980, p. 84) discuss propositional meanings as idea-units composed of two parts: "the judgement, or *predicate*, and one or more objects, or *arguments*." Predicates involve judgments or attributes of objects or happenings (*big* boy, *happy* times, *on* the table); arguments entail the number of propositions or idea-units (*The big boy had the hammer* and *hit the nail*). Neither the judgment (predicate) nor the argument (proposition) has a simple or static relationship to sentence structure. For example, predicates can be expressed as prepositions, adverbs, adjectives, conjunctions and so forth.

Multiple and figurative meanings of words represent an intriguing link between referential and propositional content. Interpreting and using multiple meanings of words require sophisticated use of symbols and also depend on the entire context in which the utterance is used. Broad definitions of words, involving shifting frames of reference and semantic category, allow for differing interpretations of the same word. However, the semantic and syntactic contexts provide the references for determining the word meaning. (Wiig and Semel, 1980). For example, "The water is *running*" conjures up an entirely different image from "The boy is *running*" or "The car is *running*." The use of figurative language by preschoolers and older children is sometimes amusing and occurs frequently in everyday speech ("sad as a spanking", "hot as a firecracker", "dirty as a pig").

Johnston and Kamhi (1980) reported their study of semantic complexity in the speech of language-impaired children and younger, MLU-matched (same number of morphemes-per-utterance) children and noted that language-impaired children expressed fewer propositions per utterance with fewer adverbial and modifying expressions. The authors interpreted the data as descriptive of language-impaired children in the following ways:

1. Language-impaired children are more likely than normal speakers to express items referring to the present and the observable.
2. Language-impaired children experience difficulty with the processes of utterance formulation.
3. Language-impaired children exhibit difficulty with the production of language patterns involving formal features distinct from direct ties to meaning (for example, qualifiers and expansions of meaning).

Wiig and Semel (1976; 1980) categorize language production in terms of divergent and convergent abilities. They describe convergent language problems as difficulties experienced when semantic constraints (word selection requirements) and linguistic constraints (such as grammatical forms) are placed on the speaker. Linguistic constraints determine the structural aspects of the message; semantic constraints determine the meaning to be expressed with the best words for that message. According to Wiig and Semel, children with convergent production disabilities have difficulty with word finding, specific answers to questions, and fill-in-the-blank tasks, as well as difficulty with defining words or providing explanations. They suggest that children with divergent production disabilities may not be able to express a variety of solutions to problems, have difficulty expanding a topic, or have trouble discussing items of their own choosing. In pragmatic terms, however, the divergent production problems described by Wiig and Semel could indicate a deficiency in language *use*. The inability to produce solutions to problems or to expand a topic could reflect underdeveloped language function or communication acts. Some language-deficient children excel when the constraints of semantic and linguistic requirements are removed (for example, questions requiring specific answers). They may be able to elaborate in fluent and original ways, although they ramble without restraining their own verbosity when no external controls are imposed.

Assessment of Expressive Language Content:
Quantitative Methods

Because content, or semantics, overlaps other language components of form and use, many assessment devices include both syntactic and semantic tasks. For example, tasks requiring a child to complete a sentence with the most appropriate word also require some knowledge of the grammatical system. Some quantifying measures designed to assess semantic aspects of language production include the following:

1. *ITPA:* Auditory Association subtest (Kirk, McCarthy, and Kirk, 1968). Requires the child to finish a sentence with one word that expresses the verbal analogy projected in the sentence
2. *Detroit Tests of Learning Aptitude:* Verbal Opposites subtest (Baker and Leland, 1967). Asks child for opposites to the simulus words
3. *ITPA:* Verbal Expression subtest (Kirk, McCarthy, and Kirk, 1968). Asks child to describe the characteristics of four common objects
4. *Detroit Tests of Learning Aptitude:* Free Association subtest (Baker and Leland, 1967). A timed task requiring the child to produce any words he can think of
5. *Type-token ratio* (Templin, 1957). A procedure for determining vocabulary usage based on the number of different words produced in a 50-utterance sample, the total number of words produced in the sample, and a ratio derived from these numbers

Assessment of Expressive Language Content:
Qualitative Methods

Language formation and production problems in language-impaired children may be severe and obvious to the most casual observer, or they may be subtle enough to be overlooked in educational and remediation plans. Some characteristics of expressive disorders in children with content (semantic) disorders can be observed in their spontaneous speech. These characteristics, which somewhat overlap observations of form and use, include the following:

1. *Use of a large number of words combined with semantically incomplete or incorrect utterances.* For example, there may be limitations in the expression of time, space, or number relationships.
"He got six fish and five and twelve"
"He eat"
2. *Oversimplification of ideas that could be formulated more succinctly.*
"I want to go"
"I want to go home"
"I want to see Mom"
"I want to hug Mom"
3. *Difficulty with word finding.* Some children must attempt to describe what they want when they fail to retrieve the appropriate word. Even then, their descriptions may be inadequate.

Clinician	*Child*
What do you want?	I want the catcher thing . . . you know. . . .
What's that?	For the ball in it . . . and . . . a thing. . . .
To catch a ball with?	Yeah, um . . .
What's it called?	Uh . . . a hand catch thing. . . .

4. *Misuse of words for the situation.* Language-deficient children often have difficulty using semantically complex relations and choose semantic forms which are slightly inaccurate.

Clinician	Child
Where did you go?	To *take* a haircut.
Did your brother go?	Yeah, he went to take a haircut, too.

5. *Inappropriate word combinations for conveying information.* Some children seem to have difficulty with the semantic and syntactic combinations they need to convey a message appropriately:

Clinician	Child
What do you want?	I want the thing that plays.
What do you mean?	The mitt plays. *(asking for the baseball mitt)*

6. *Difficulty defining words.* The school-age child should be able to define single-meaning and multiple-meaning words.

7. *Trouble explaining metaphors, adages, similes, and other figurative uses of speech.* Young school-age children usually can provide some explanation of figurative uses of speech, though they may not be very precise.

The stilted and inflexible language production of some language-deficient children with disorders of content takes many forms. Lucas (1980, pp. 86–87) notes that the disruption of word use and selection interferes with a child's communicative effectiveness. She provides a set of questions for the clinician to consider in determining a child's expressive semantic and pragmatic abilities. Those most pertinent to semantic disorders are as follows:

1. Does the child express objects, actions, and events in a variety of (semantic) relationships?
2. Does the child spontaneously generate new utterances in new contexts?
3. Does the child use similar semantic combinations over and over to the exclusion of other combinations?
4. Does the child use a variety of qualifiers and descriptors such as terms of time, space, and amount?

Miller (1981) describes a nonstandardized procedure for analyzing the range of a child's vocabulary called a "semantic field analysis." Semantic field analysis facilitates study of the diversity and complexity of a child's vocabulary in terms of number of different meaning categories, as well as different words within categories. It also allows the investigation of spatial and temporal relations, which Miller notes can be indicative of discrepancies between notions the child can only conceive and those he/she can actually describe.

Word selection and word combination deficiencies can be difficult to describe in either highly verbal children or children with low verbal output. Limitations of content in the language-impaired child require that the clinician assess the child's production skills in all the various ways and situations that might produce adequate quantitative and qualitative information for determining the child's intervention needs.

Expressive Deficiencies of Form Language form refers to the linguistic structure of utterances, including pronunciation, articulation, word and sound sequencing, use of grammatical rules, structural complexity and adequacy, sentence types, and grammatical morphemes. Language-disabled children and adolescents exhibit deficits in the acquisition and/or use of both morphology and syntax (Johnson and Myklebust, 1967; Vogel, 1974; Wiig and Semel, 1976; Menyuk, 1969). Some studies indicate that the spontaneous production of syntax in some language-deficient children may not differ from that of academic achievers during spontaneous conversation, but differences appear in structured tasks of sentence repetition or sentence completion (Rosenthal, 1970; Vogel, 1974; Wiig and Semel, 1976). It is possible that some language-disabled children compensate for language deficits when semantic and/or linguistic constraints are minimal, such as in casual conversation. But when constraints are imposed or when they must transfer spoken language to written form, these children's linguistic abilities may prove inadequate.

Delays in the acquisition and use of morphology and syntax in spoken language may persist through the primary grades and into even higher grades. Vogel (1974) compared the syntactic and morphological abilities of 20 children experiencing reading deficiencies with 20 normal children, using the *Northwestern Syntax Screening Test (NSST)* (Lee, 1969). The children, ranging from seven and one-half to eight and one-half years old, showed no significant differences in the oral expressive syntax portion, although no analysis was performed of the same structures in written form. However, in 1975 Wiig and Semel used the NSST with 34 language-deficient children and 17 high academic achievers from 7 to 11 years old. The language-deficient children had significant delays in the comprehension of syntactic structures. Wiig and Semel (1975) also reported a study in which they observed learning-disabled adolescents on sentence production tasks. The adolescents produced significantly more agrammatical and incomplete sentences than their peers who were achieving on grade level.

Although word order is considered one of the earliest devices by which children convey information before they acquire morphological markers (Bloom, 1970), word order is not always correctly observed by language-impaired children. Berry (1969) and Menyuk (1964; 1969) provide examples of speech that they consider deviant in word order. For example,

Berry's list (p. 231) of misordered sentences spoken by a six-year-old boy
with serious language problems includes the following:

> "Look me no."
>
> "Me buy go candy."
>
> "He school no go Saturday."
>
> "Lost mittens me."

Clearly these versions of word order are not typical of a normal young
child's immature constructions.

If young language-impaired children do not observe word order as an
indicator of semantic and syntactic relationships, they may fail to acquire the
necessary grammatical and morphological forms for higher-level language
situations demanding more complex linguistic distinctions (Berry, 1969;
Bloom, 1978).

Development of complex phonological, morphological, and grammatical
systems provides the vehicle for utterances to become functionally complex
so that the speaker can convey more than one meaning at a time (Halliday,
1973). Language-deficient children often do not attain these complexities.
Johnston and Kamhi (1980) reported that the language-impaired children
in their study encoded different meanings in their utterances, but they
displayed less grammatical facility than the normal children with equivalent
utterance length.

The construction of either oral or written complex sentences seems difficult for many school-age language-impaired children. Sentence complexity
is determined by the presence of more than one main verb. Miller (1981)
describes two classes of complex sentences:

1. *Conjoined sentences*—sentences composed of more than one full sentence
   with the utterances joined by a conjunction (and, but, after, and the rest.)
2. *Embedded sentences*—sentences with a sentencelike segment containing a
   main verb within a larger sentence. Miller cites the following types of embed-
   cing:
   a. Simple infinitive clauses (I'll get the book *to read*)
   b. Propositional complements (I said *that you can do it*)
   c Relative clauses (Look at the good story *that I wrote*)
   d Gerund clauses (Look at her *running around the track*)
   e. Double embeddings (I can *do it myself now*)

Miller also describes sentences that demonstrate both conjoined and embedded clauses within one utterance (He had to go with us, *because* it was
too hot to walk.).

One type of structural disorder associated with language-impaired children is the expression of grammatical morphemes. Grammatical morphemes are discussed here as an example of the many structural complexities of language that many language-deficient children do not develop adequately.

Morphology and syntax are two subsystems of grammar (Winitz, 1966). Morphology encompasses the rules describing inflections and derivations of words; syntax consists of the rules determining the ordering of words into sentences. Brown (1973, pp. 11–12) states that morphemes modulate meaning and distinguishes between basic content and modulations of content.

> One easily conceives of meanings for naming words (nouns, verbs, and adjectives) in the absence of any modulation but one does not easily conceive of number, past tense, progressive aspect, referent specificity, and the like, in abstraction from any thing, person, action, state, or quality.

English grammatical morphemes often are redundant; it is linguistically obligatory to provide morphemes in the utterance, even if the meaning is semantically redundant. (For example, the plural marker *s* is required linguistically in the sentence "Two boy__run," even though plurality has been indicated by the word "two" and the addition of the plural *s* is a redundant indication of plurality.) Redundancies may be necessary for dealing with the complexities of language. The simplest grammar, which would convey all meanings with the fewest rules and exclude all redundancies, might not be the most efficient for the rapid and continuous interchange of speech (Menyuk, 1969). In English, the redundant indications of plurality or tense [A (singular) girl (singular) runs (singular).] allow the listener to rapidly scan the message for meaning without being forced to attend to every word spoken.

Redundancy may be a primary factor in the inadequate development of morphemes in some language-deficient children. The normal child learns adult rules for appropriate omission of grammatical forms, such as elliptical utterances. Language-impaired children continue to omit linguistically obligatory morphemes, even though their utterances increase in length and semantic complexity.

> "Two boy run."
>
> "Momma hat all dirty."
>
> "Them didn't runned faster than the mices."

The semantic function of morphemes is not usually considered in the remediation of linguistic form, although literature indicates that meaning influences morphological forms used by children (Bloom, 1970; Slobin,

1971; Brown, 1973; Bowerman, 1978). The function of morphemes as modulators of meaning has been minimized in some studies that utilize distributional analyses of morphemes or that classify morphemes only according to parts of speech. The classification of morphemes solely as grammatical units prohibits the study of semantic influences on errors and may camouflage important information concerning the rules governing morpheme production. To understand errors in morpheme production, it is necessary to consider some of the grammatical and semantic components involved and then apply this understanding to analysis of language samples.

Morphemes acquire their meaning from the information they signal. Prepositions are linguistic structures that specify in the surface structure of utterances basic semantic concepts that are part of the deep structure of utterances. For example, certain English prepositions indicate location (*in* the box, *on* the table, *under* the chair, *at* the store, *to* the park). The semantic concept of instrument is signaled by the prepositions *with* and *by* (Hit it *with* the hammer. He was cut *by* the knife.) and signal a cause-and-effect proposition between an action and an object. *To* and *for* mark semantic concepts labeled as benefactive and signal the beneficiary or recipient of some act or process (Give it *to* me. Buy the present *for* her.). A preposition also can function as an indicator of the semantic concept of accompaniment (Go *with* me).

Other grammatical morphemes modulate basic meanings of an utterance. Among these are nouns inflected for plurality (I have some shoe*s*.) and irregular plurals, including changes of the stem noun (See the *mice*). The possessor-possessed relation between two nouns, which is already marked by word order, is further signaled by possessive inflections (Daddy'*s* chair), and possessive pronouns (*my* chair).

It is necessary to consider semantic function as well as grammatic form so that rules governing incorrect production of morphemes can be identified. For example, the lexical item "to" cannot be considered solely a grammatical form, because the meaning, signaled by the word and the functions it serves, varies with the context of the utterance.

The same word *(to)* can serve as a locative preposition, a marker of the semantic role of beneficiary, a verb particle (Listen *to* me.), or part of a colloquial expression (Go *to* sleep.).

Lexical Item	Grammatical Form	Semantic Feature
to ("I go *to* town.")	preposition	location marker (subcategory of directionality)
to ("Give it *to* her.")	preposition	benefactive marker of semantic role of beneficiary

Analysis of language behavior, whether qualitative or quantitative, should consider both form and meaning of language. Apparently both grammatical construction and semantic role affect morpheme acquisition in early language, and a discrepancy between the acquisition of grammatical form and semantic function in a language-impaired child may offer valuable information for assessment and for remediation. The growing child's expanding experiences and concepts broaden his/her meanings, forcing his/her grammar to become more complex in order to express the broader meanings. Developing complex grammatical systems is a means of coordinating different communicative intents so that expressions can become more useful. A child with language dysfunctions may not develop each component of language with uniform competence, and may experience interruption of some aspect of communication. For example, a child may develop adequate semantic roles but not have the syntactic or morphological structures necessary for conveying information in conventional linguistic form.

Clinician	Child	Interpretation of Utterance
What happens to kids at your school when they get into trouble?	Have sit down.	They have to sit down.
Is that all?	Sometime a teacher see. see. Have a talk.	Sometimes the teacher sees them and they have a talk.
The teacher sees them?	Have a talk.	They have a talk.

Assessing speech and language skills of language-impaired children must not exclude one component of language in the measurement of another.

Assessment of Expressive Language Form: Quantitative Methods

There are several devices for assessing spontaneous or elicited speech forms in language-impaired children. Morehead and Ingram (1973) determine linguistic level by the mean number of morphemes per utterance and use this criterion for matching normal and language-deviant groups rather than general developmental criteria. Roger Brown (1970; 1973) indicated that the mean number of morphemes per utterance is a reliable indicator of linguistic level, because the mean length of utterance (MLU) is an excellent simple index of grammatical development. Other studies (Shriner, 1969; Leonard, 1972; Olson, 1972; Davis and Seitz 1975) indicate that the level of language development is reflected more accurately in a young speaker by mean-length utterance than age. MLU is calculated by dividing the total number of morphemes in a series of utterances by the number of utterances.

As a young child's language increases in number and complexity of syntactic and semantic rules, the length of utterances increases until he/she reaches a sophisticated language level of embedding clauses. This then reduces the length of utterances although they may be very complex grammatically (Wiig and Semel, 1980; Miller, 1981). As a child reaches three and one-half to four, the effectiveness of MLU as a sensitive quantitative measure begins to decrease. Cazden (1972) indicates that there is a greater density of ideas in a single sentence as the child develops. Hass and Wettman (1974) and Lucas (1980) also report an increase in embedding with age, reducing the number of morphemes produced in a complex utterance. ("He has five dogs and three dogs and we saw them" = 13 morphemes; "We saw his five dogs" = 6 morphemes.)

Another method of language sample analysis is the *Developmental Sentence Scoring DSS* developed by Lee (1974). It measures structural complexity, particularly of verb forms. The DSS supplies additional qualitative data on frequency and type of constructions used in noun modifiers, personal pronouns, conjunctions, and interrogatives.

Chapman (1978) discusses a structural analysis procedure for analyzing a child's simple utterances by major structural categories.

1. Fourteen grammatical morphemes (after Brown, 1973)
2. Active, affirmative, declarative sentences
3. Negatives
4. Yes/no questions
5. Wh-questions, and complex sentences, including embedded and conjoined utterances.

Through the use of structural development charts containing criteria for "Assignment of Structural Stage," Chapman indicates six types of structural forms for analysis.

1. Single-word utterances
2. Noun-phrase elaboration
3. Verb-phrase elaboration
4. Negation
5. Yes/no questions
6. Wh-questions

Data from the structural development charts help determine the stage for each structural development.

Paul's (1980) complex-sentence development charts describe advances in the development of complex sentence production. He suggests at least five items to look for when analyzing free speech production.

1. Percentage of true complex sentences within the speech sample
2. Forms of embedding (for instance, simple infinitive clauses, relative clauses)
3. Forms of conjoined sentences
4. Appearance of specific conjunctions
5. Average number of different conjunctions

Complex-sentence analysis can be performed with the *"Assigning Structural Stage"* procedure described by Chapman or it can be used separately. Other procedures that provide information regarding a child's structural proficiencies include the following:

1. *ITPA*: Grammatic Closure sub-test (Kirk, McCarthy, and Kirk, 1968)
   A sentence-completion test designed to evaluate a child's application of grammatical rules to plurals, possessives, tenses, adverbs, prepositions, comparatives, and pronouns
2. *Northwestern Syntax Screening:* Expressive sub-test (Lee, 1969)
   Requires verbatim repetition of grammatical structures within sentences
3. *Carrow Elicited Language Inventory* (Carrow, 1974)
   Determines a child's use of grammatical structures through sentence imitation

Whatever combinations of qualitative and quantitative strategies are used in language assessment, it is important to deal with all components of the language system and its use. Using one method, such as quantitative analysis, to the exclusion of another method, can mask important information regarding the child's language. Behavioral observations should be weighed with test data when making clinical judgments of impaired language functioning. When a discrepancy occurs between test data and clinical opinion, the clinician must decide which index to weigh more heavily (Allen, Bliss, and Timmons, 1981).

Assessment of Expressive Language Form: Qualitative
Methods

Qualitative analysis of spontaneous utterances can aid in describing linguistic rules employed by language-disordered children, because structural and semantic rule patterns vary with the type and severity of the disorder. For example, a child with semantic problems may rely on a different set of rules for production from the child with syntactical problems. Normal speakers learn to construct their utterances by acquiring and applying rules of the language system (for example, phonology, syntax, semantics, and communicative interactions). Language development involves appropriate specificity and generalization of rules and their applications. Menyuk (1969) and Weiner (1974) suggest that language-deviant children form hypotheses about language that interfere with language refinement and sophistication. Menyuk suggests that deficient speakers acquire certain patterns and then reach plateaus, failing to continue the refinement of language subsystems. Overgeneralizations occur when a child develops early rules for form and function before learning all the linguistic representations necessary for sophisticated language production. For example, a young child might overgeneralize a grammatical rule (+ ed = past, therefore: "Today I go." "Yesterday I goed.").

A language-impaired child sometimes does not learn exceptions to the rules of language, as a normally-developing child does. In Menyuk's terms generalization of a language rule becomes a dead-end for the child who does not advance to specific rules for certain forms. It seems that the dead-end rule applies to other components of language in language-impaired children. Literal interpretation of word meaning may indicate underspecification of word category and use; spelling errors may represent overgeneralization of phonetic patterns. Oversimplification of language system components seems to restrict high-level development in many language-impaired children. This phenomenon appears to occur in one component (grammar) and not in another (semantics) in some language-deficient children. Therefore, one component of language may be well developed while another is deficient.

Spontaneous language samples may have an advantage over other methods of language sampling in qualitative analysis (Lucas, 1980; Wiig and Semel, 1980). They seem to place fewer constraints on the child than such structured evaluation devices as imitation or elicited utterances. Prutting, Gallagher, and Mulac (1975) indicate that children may produce syntactic structures in spontaneous speech that are not evident in elicited language samples. A child may imitate more complex utterances than he/she can produce spontaneously, although this extended production does not necessarily indicate his/her level of competence (Lucas, 1980). According to Lucas (p. 20) "direct imitation . . . does not have a one-to-one correspondence with the child's spontaneous skills."

Bloom (1970) reported substantial qualitative differences between spontaneous and elicited utterances. Grammatical forms that had occurred spontaneously often did not occur in response to questions that might be expected to elicit the same form. The similarities between repeated and spontaneous utterances may not be the same for deviant-speaking children and normal children (Menyuk, 1969; Menyuk and Looney, 1972), and assessment tools using imitation may not provide the same information about language-deviant children that they provide about normal children. Most studies using imitation in evaluation have examined syntax and have provided little information about the role of imitation in the development of semantic abilities. In a study comparing the *Northwestern Syntax Screening Test (NSST) (Lee, 1969) to a spontaneous language sample, Prutting, Gallagher, and Mulac (1975) noted that a child may fail to produce a grammatical distinction on the NSST but correctly produce that distinction in spontaneous speech.*

USING CONTEXT IN QUALITATIVE ANALYSIS. Children learn language in context, with utterances rarely occurring in isolation or conveying meaning in isolation (Wallach and Lee, 1980). The study of isolated utterances should be only one part of language analysis. Although some studies have focused on a single word or a morphological form without including the complete utterance spontaneously produced by the child (Kirk, McCarthy, and Kirk, 1968; Lee and Canter, 1971), a large sample of spontaneous, or "free," speech may be more representative of the full range of production (Tyack, 1972; Brown, 1973; Morehead and Ingram, 1973; Bloom, 1978 Miller, 1981). Complete samples of a child's utterances would produce valuable information about his/her productions. Usually the reliability of a measure increases as the size of the sample behavior is increased. For example, Johnson and Tomblin (1976) estimated reliability for "Developmental Sentence Scoring" as determined by sample size and concluded that the "estimated reliability values increased for all scoring categories as the sample size increased" (p. 377). A representative sample should be enough to provide good examples of the child's productive competencies. Opinions regarding the size of the sample vary. Lucas (1980) suggests a minimum of 50 utterances, but acknowledges that in low verbal children 25 utterances may have to suffice. Tyack (1972) suggests a minimum of 100 utterances, while Wood (1976) used 500 spontaneous, interpretable utterances for analysis. Lucas (1980) and Miller (1981) describe materials and contexts for obtaining samples from children of various ages, along with goals for qualitative analysis.

Utterance interpretation, essential for analysis of errors, can be difficult with the distorted speech of some language-impaired children. However, as Bloom (1970) suggests, interpretation is often enhanced by consideration of contextual and situational information. For example, some language-deficient children omit grammatical forms in their utterances. However, the utterances are still interpretable in many instances because the omitted forms are semantically redundant, and the meaning is still clear to the listener. Bloom indicated that if the semantic function of the utterance is not interpreted, speech analysis is confined to linguistic descriptions of the form of speech. Although some utterances are uninterpretable or ambiguous, many are interpretable through observations of the context, the child's behaviors, and the situation. Analysis of the child's additions, substitutions (distortions), and/or omissions of structural form can be performed with this interpretation. Table 2–4 lists examples of utterance interpretation.

Selecting structures for analysis should be partly based on regular occurrence of the item in the child's speech. For example, Leonard (1972) did not include a structure for analysis unless it occurred two or more times in the child's speech. Bloom (1970) established criteria to determine regularities of performance that "could be used as evidence for inferring the most productive and stable components of underlying competence" (p. 17). Bloom's criteria involved considering a structure unique if it occurred only once in the speech sample, marginal if it occurred fewer than five times, and productive (rule-based) if it occurred five or more times. Selection of utterances for analysis usually involves disregarding ambiguous or uninterpretable utterances.

Lucas (1980) suggests questions to apply to the analysis of speech samples. Adaptation of these questions to the analysis of linguistic form include:

1. Does the child use similar syntactic constructions over and over to the exclusion of various other constructions?
2. Are there obvious indications of disorders of grammar, word order, or phonology?
3. Does the child generate new (forms of) utterances in new contexts? (For more on this, see the section on function.)

Whatever approaches are used in the assessment of production in language-impaired children, analyses should result in a description of the child's production patterns and an attempt to determine the rules reflected in the descriptions.

receptive deficiencies: description and assessment

As indicated earlier, the term receptive deficiencies identifies inadequate interpretation of spoken or written language input in terms of attaching significance to the input, interpreting grammatical constructions, recognizing sounds or letters, understanding word meanings, and understanding relationships expressed in language. As with expressive deficiencies, receptive deficiencies are discussed in terms of use, content, and form of the recipient's native language.

It has been commonly accepted that comprehension precedes production; however, this assumption warrants more scrutiny with both normal speakers and language-impaired children (Nelson, 1981). Vygotsky (1962) indicates that production can precede comprehension developmentally, at least for some cognitively difficult functions, and de Villiers and de Villiers (1978) suggest that children monitor their own speech for accuracy before

TABLE 2–4

Examples of Utterance Interpretation

STIMULUS	RESPONSE	INTERPRETATION
What?	I drive in car. Play in a sand. Then I play in a rocket. That all. Then play in mud, too.	I drive in a car. I play in the sand. That's all. Then I play in mud too.
Did you go on a field trip?	I going to a fire station. Then I going to a mail place.	I went to a fire station. Then I went to a mail place.
Tell her about your trip to the fire station.	I went somewhere. And Mother say on that one I can't go. I got chicken pox. And I didn't go on a trip. I can't go. I got chicken pox.	And mother said I couldn't go on that one. I had chicken pox. And I didn't go on the trip.
Tell her about your trip to the fire station. What?	I went to a fire station. There a fire, real quick he put on his boots. Put on his firehat. Then he go for a fire.	If there's a fire he puts on his boots real quick. He puts on his firehat. Then he goes to a fire.
Do you have a pool at your house? (child says water is out of pool) How can you swim if there's no water? I'd be mad, too.	It's broken. We got all mad. I mad at that swimming pool.	I'm mad at that swimming pool.
(child takes gum out of her pocket) Huh? (child unwraps gum and holds paper) I'll throw it away in just a minute. (E puts wrapper in her purse) (child mashes and hits gum before putting it in her mouth) What did you do that to your gum for? Oh! (child points to gum in her mouth) What did you say? You do? If you don't like hot gum, I'll try to get you a different kind of gum.	I gonna open it. Can I open it? Is there a garbage? That's a garbage? I was fixing it. It's hot. It's hot. I don't like. It's hot.	I'm gonna open it. Is that a garbage? I don't like it.
(making turning movement with her hands) The bowl? Why? Oh! (child indicates she helps her mother stir the cake)	You just turn round. It stop and won't go.	You just turn it around. It stops and won't go.

TABLE 2–4 continued

STIMULUS	RESPONSE	INTERPRETATION
Then what do you do after you turn it around and mix it up?	Then you put ice on there.	Then you put icing on there.
What were you telling me about your refrigerator? Oh!	We put it refrigerator.	We put it in the refrigerator.
	We got three refrigerator. Two's a old. One's kitchen's old. They got beer in's old too. One's kinda dirty. One's clean.	We have three refrigerators. Two are old. The one in the kitchen is old. The one they got beer in is old, too.
You put the stuff in the refrigerator and then what?	You wait to the dining room and wait. Somebody get it.	You wait in the dining room and wait for somebody to get it.

they are aware that they are applying language in an analytical way. The sequence of acquisition of receptive/expressive skills in language is not to be argued here, but the interrelatedness of reception and expression is obvious. Language-impaired children demonstrate deficiencies, as well as adequacies, of reception and expression, and assessment and intervention should not exclude either reception or expression. Discussion of the components of receptive deficiencies, will not reiterate that of expressive deficiencies; it will only note areas that seem primarily related to receptive disorders that were not examined before. Assessment and analysis should investigate the assumption that any deficient area in a child's speech production might have a counterpart in the child's speech reception.

Inadequate reception of any aspects of communication interferes with normal communicative interaction and can impede learning. A child who does not receive or comprehend the complete message may fail to acquire new information, have difficulty learning in group situations, misinterpret a speaker's intention, or have trouble understanding multiple meanings of words. Some children have such severe receptive disorders they understand the message only if provided with supportive visual clues like gestures or pictures. If some children miss a part of the message because of background noise, they seem unable to determine the missing form to complete the message for themselves. For example, "Go get a (cough)-cil and paper." If a child does not recognize the entire message, then the response may be dependent on separate items within the utterance.

Teachers and parents describe their observations of receptive language disorders as follows:

"He just doesn't mind."

"Sometimes he acts like he's looking right through me when I tell him something. Why doesn't he answer?"

"I know he can hear, because he hates loud noises and covers his ears when the vacuum cleaner is on. But sometimes I would swear he only hears me when he's looking at me."

"I have to tell her everything ten times and even show her what I want before anything registers. But she learns some things so fast; she never gets lost, and she can paint or draw anything she sees."

"He never answers the question I ask him."

Receptive Deficiencies of Use Inadequate reception of *use* refers to the misunderstanding or misinterpretation of the intended message. Inadequate reception includes:

1. *difficulty interpreting direct and indirect speech acts, including the "reading" of verbal and nonverbal devices (that is, integrating the intent, content, and form of the utterance to interpret the message).* This is related to perlocutionary force, which is the effect that utterances have on the listener (for instance, persuasion, conviction).
2. *difficulty participating as a conversational partner by providing appropriate responses to the topic and the situation.* A person also gives the speaker adequate feedback regarding the conversation (asking for clarification, and so on).

Success in these behaviors requires the interaction of use, content, and form; often the listener must interpret the form and content in which a message is framed in order to interpret the message. *Metalinguistic skills* are integral to the success of language interpretation. In Halliday's (1977) terms it appears that the child must have full cognizance of the pragmatic and mathetic functions of language to appropriately interpret input. Ways in which language-impaired children have difficulty interpreting direct and indirect speech acts include the following:

1. *Tendency to be concrete and literal.* Language-impaired children often do not recognize the presuppositional information available in prior content, focusing their attention on the surface meaning of separate words. This results in the overly literal interpretation of utterances, including idioms, similes, adages, and metaphors.

Clinician	*Child*
Now we have a secret. Don't let the cat out of the bag.	Oh! Can he breathe?

2. *Difficulty understanding cause-and-effect relationships.* The child must interpret the potential meaning of, and predict the consequences of, actions described. The problem is apparent when the language-impaired child is asked to interpret stories, predict the outcome of events, or understand absurdities.

Clinician	*Child*
I heard about a man who walked in the woods two times, and the first time he got lost and died. . . .	
Why doesn't that story make sense?	I guess he should have gotten a compass.

The child's failure to attend to preceding information in the utterance, even though the vocabulary is well within his/her grasp, may show an inability to recognize the combinatorial meaning of the words (receptive disorder of *content*) as well as poor use of prior information (receptive disorder of *use*). Wiig and Semel (1980) illustrate inadequate interpretation of utterances in which the child must attend to the compositional meaning of words, demonstrating the child's failure to recognize such *presuppositional* clues as world knowledge and information from preceding utterances. Their example notes various ways in which the child is told it may rain and he/she should grasp the implied, unspoken message (depending on the speaker and the situation). For example:

a. it may not rain (world knowledge: when it's cloudy, it doesn't always rain) (previous context "may")
b. wear a raincoat (shared knowledge: what Mother always says when it rains)
c. come inside to stay dry (listener specific knowledge: hating to get wet)

3. *Misinterpretation of indirect or polite forms of conversation.* Frequently language-impaired children do not interpret the intent of the message if it is conveyed through indirect forms, nor do they pay attention to nonverbal information (situational clues) like facial expression, word emphasis, or implied speaker needs

Adult	*Child*
Can you open the door? *(with an armful of groceries)*	Yes I can. I'm very strong. *(without moving from chair)*

An interview with a sixteen year-old boy who had been seriously language deficient as a young child illustrates the conversational inadequacies of a person who talks but does not participate adequately as a communication partner:

Interviewer	*Adolescent*
Can you drive a car?	Yes, I can drive a car.
What color is your car?	My car is green.
Too bad it's not orange and white, *(the young man's school colors)* so you can drive it to school.	Is it too bad?
I mean it would be nice if your car were the same colors as your school colors.	Oh!
Do you like to zip around in it?	No, I do not like to.
What do you like to do with it?	I like to drive it.

Would you like to have some of this? *(pointing to coke on the table)*	Yes, I would. *(making no movement)*
You may have it. *(extending coke to him)*	Thank you. *(no movement)*
Take the coke, and drink it.	All right. *(takes coke and drinks it)*

The young man's ability to construct grammatically adequate utterances is apparent. It appears he had been taught to respond to the content of a question but not to interpret the intent of utterances on the basis of their compositional meaning, nor to attend to contextual or world information in interpreting utterances. He apparently did not understand the intent of some of the indirect speech acts directed to him ("Would you like to have some of this?"); in other situations, his misinterpretations could be mistaken for smart-aleck retorts. He did not interpret "would you?" or "don't you?" as indirect forms of request or instruction; nor did he understand word substitutions by their contextually defined use (zip/drive); nor did he interpret the intent of the nonverbal message (gestures with the coke).

Oversimplification or inadequate interpretation of the pragmatic rules of conversation often is characteristic of language-deficient children. Their misunderstanding of communicative intent and their failure to incorporate situational clues into their interpretation of the message can result in social conflict.

Teacher	*Child*
	(standing in front of chalkboard between class and board)
John, the children can't see the board	Oh, what's the matter with their eyes?

Parents often describe their language-impaired child's inadequate interpretation of conversation with sadness and frustration:

> She always has her feelings hurt, because she thinks people are making fun of her when they joke. She never knows what we "mean" when we explain that people like her and that's why they play by making jokes.

Deficiencies in word interpretation do not stop with literacy or advancement through school. A colleague teaching in a local college related this story about a student (who *must* have been one of my language-impaired children from previous years of therapy):

> A journalism class at the college was given a test that included a question that asked why afternoon newspapers around the country were folding. The student wrote, "folding is easier than rolling them and putting rubberbands around them."

The difficulties language-impaired children experience in *participating as a conversation partner* include the following:

> *Misunderstanding of turn taking in conversation, games, and classroom participation.* The language-deficient child frequently acts as though the other partners in the conversation, game, or discussion have no bearing on his/her utterances or actions. The language-impaired child may not pay attention to what is said, when it is said, or or how it is said. In this way, language-impaired children do not maintain the topic of conversation and offer utterances that seem very incoherent to the listener.
>
> *Difficulty repairing communication breakdowns.* Many language-impaired children may not understand that they have misinterpreted the message, or may not recognize that they must inform the speaker of needed clarification or repetition. When the speaker delivers a message, the language-deficient child may respond with a nod or "um hum," relinquishing the conversational turn to the speaker and avoiding an answer. The speaker may not know what the child did not understand, or even that there is any confusion about the message.

Communication breakdowns occur frequently with language-deficient children, not only because they do not understand the words, but because they do not know how to attend to the entire package of communicative information, and they do not signal the speaker about a misinterpretation of the message.

Assessment of Receptive Language Use

At the time of this writing, no standardized measure of the reception of language use is available. Clinical observation of children's interpretations of utterances can be adapted from some of the questions and criterion-referenced assessment tools discussed in the section on expressive uses of language. Questions that may help the clinician analyze receptive use of language include the following:

1. Does the child respond to verbal input intended to serve a variety of communicative functions (for instance, responding to indirect forms of request)?
2. Does the child interpret nonverbal and situational clues?
3. Does the child interpret utterances whose meaning requires integration with the previous context or shared speaker/listener information?
4. Dces the child respond to paralinguistic clues (such as prosody, gestures, and eye contact)?
5. Does the child respond to new information presented verbally in a way that seems to be incorporated into the child's store of knowledge (for example, using language for learning)?

Receptive uses of language for interaction and learning can be limited in language-deficient children and can interfere with their personal and social development as well as their academic achievement. The interaction of language use, content, and form makes it difficult to ascertain the precise area of receptive breakdown in language-impaired children. Precision of diagnosis in that sense is not as important as the inclusion of all components of language in the assessment process.

Receptive Deficiencies of Content   Reception of language content includes interpreting the meaning of individual words and word combinations in both oral and written utterances, and includes both *referential* and *propositional* aspects of meaning. Referential meaning indicates categories or subcategories of word meaning; *propositional*, or compositional, meaning requires integration of word meaning with sentence and topic meaning. Normal listeners do not concentrate on one sentence at a time because sentence sequences ordinarily are semantically integrated and listeners respond to the total message. That is, the comprehension of content requires the integration of information across sentences into the total theme along with inferences made by the listener (Dale, 1976; Clark and Haviland, 1977; Stark and Wallach 1980). Comprehension of content also demands that the listener relate new information to prior context and information (Bransford and Nitsch, 1978; Kail and Marshall, 1978). Integration of content with prior information was discussed in the sections on expressive and receptive use of language.

Comprehension is not a passive act; it demands participation from the listener/reader. Older children and adults use their semantic knowledge to fill gaps in information and integrate utterances into unified meaning (Dale, 1976; Blachowicz, 1977–78). Some older, language-impaired children respond to utterances with limited meanings for words, without responding to the composite meaning of the utterance. Receptive disorders of content can include both referential and propositional disorders of meanings, some of which are described in the next section.

Receptive Disorders of Referential Meaning

Language-impaired children often are restricted in their interpretation of word meaning. They respond to words by recognizing only single meanings. They do not recognize multiple meanings or subcategories of meanings, relational or descriptive terms, or expressions of speaker perspective. For example, they exhibit the following limitations:

1. Single and specific application of word meaning (see understanding of metaphors in this section)

Adult	*Child*
That was a tough job, wasn't it?	Tough? Were you chewing something?

2. Underdevelopment of relational words

Adult   *Child*
That's a tall man.   No. He's skinny, but he's *long*.

3. Misunderstanding of words that should convey the perspective of the speaker (as in deictic expressions)

Adult   *Child*

Put the pencil over here.   Over here? *(from across room)*

No, *here*, on *my* desk.
(pointing to location)   Oh! *(brings pencil)*

Receptive Disorders of Propositional Meaning

Some language-impaired children do not understand the composite meaning of utterances, including word associations within sentences, meaning relations among sentences, and influences of context and situation on meaning, as shown below:

1. Failure to consider word association within sentences (often includes recognition of both semantic and syntactic relationships)

Clinician   *Child*

Do boys eat beans?   Yes.

Do beans eat boys?   Yes. I told you!

2. Failure to consider intersentence relations

Parent   *Child*
John and I are going to town
Do you want to go?   Go where?

To town?   Who's going?

3. Failure to rely on the composite meaning of the utterance(s) to interpret the meaning

Teacher   *Child*
Let's use this for a chair
while we rest.   That's not a chair.
                                 That's a box.

Word meaning changes with context and situation, and the interpretation of utterances often depends on competence with both referential and compositional meanings. Deficiencies in both referential and compositional meanings range from severe to subtle. A severe disorder of meaning can be illustrated with the echolalic child.

Clinician	*Echolalic Child*
Do you want a coke, Johnny?	Want a coke, Johnny.
Do you want to go with your father or with your sister?	With your father or with your sister?

Even though the echolalic child's repetitions of utterances may contain perfect mimicry of syntax, morphology, and articulation, the mimicked utterances represent only a playback of sounds by the child, who does not seem to attach any meaning to them.

A more subtle disorder of meaning is represented by the child who does not understand the metaphoric meaning of utterances. Some nouns and adjectives can be used to refer to both physical and psychological properties (called dual-function words) (Gardner, Winner, Bechhofer, Wolf, 1978). For example, the word "cold" can literally describe the physical properties of ice (This ice is cold) or to characterize the personality of a person (She's cold and hard). Although competence in explaining the meaning of metaphors appears only in children as old as pre-adolescents (Winner, Rosenstiel, and Gardner, 1976), metaphoric sensitivity and understanding are discernable in early childhood and in pre-school children (Gardner, Winner, Bechhofer, Wolf, 1978). Preadolescent and adolescent language-impaired children often misinterpret metaphoric uses of utterances.

Clinician	*Adolescent*
This problem's a tough nut to crack.	Where is it? I can get it open.
His head's a shell.	Wow, I'll bet he's ugly.

Assessment of Receptive Language Content: Quantitative Methods

Some standardized measures are designed to assess a child's reception of meaning, including the following:

1. *The Peabody Picture Vocabulary Test* (Dunn, 1965)
   Requires child to indicate which of four line drawings represents a word said by the examiner
2. *Boehm Test of Basic Concepts* (Boehm, 1970)
   Measures a child's comprehension of words frequently used in early classroom instruction
3. *ITPA:* Auditory Reception subtest: (Kirk, McCarthy, and Kirk, 1968)
   Measures a child's understanding of connected utterances in noun-verb relations
4. *Detroit Tests of Learning Aptitude:* Oral Commissions subtest (Baker and Leland, 1967)
   Requires child to carry out oral instructions

5. *Test of Oral Language Development:* Picture Vocabulary: (Newcomer and Hammill, 1977)
Determines knowledge of single-word meaning in a picture identification task

6. *Toronto Tests of Receptive Vocabulary* (Toronto, 1977)
Measures understanding of vocabulary items (includes Spanish and English sections and norms)

7. *Clinical Evaluation of Language Functions:* Processing Linguistic Concepts subtest (Semel and Wiig, 1980)
Evaluates a child's ability to process, interpret and remember oral directions containing such linguistic forms as "and," "either," and "if"

8. *Clinical Evaluation of Language Functions:* Processing Relationships and Ambiguities subtest (Semel and Wiig, 1980)
Assesses the ability to process and interpret utterances with comparative terms, spatial and temporal terms, analogous relationships, metaphors, and proverbs

9. *Monroe Reading Aptitude Tests*: (Monroe, 1963)
Measures understanding of single words by identification of line drawings named by the examiner

10. *ITPA:* Auditory Association subtest (Kirk, McCarthy, and Kirk, 1968)
Assesses understanding of analogies through one word responses from child

Rizzo and Stephens (1981) compared the performance of children with normal and impaired oral language on various auditory comprehension tests. They concluded that

More than one comprehension test should be administered in an assessment program.

Inconsistencies in a child's responses (for example, on items requiring interpretation of analogies) should lead the clinician to more intensive testing. The authors recommend deep testing as discussed by Leonard, Prutting, Perozzi, and Berkley, 1978.

Assessment of Receptive Language Content: Qualitative Methods

Clinical observation of receptive language content can be based on questions that elaborate deficiencies.

1. Does the child interpret words with single and specific meaning? Does the child understand more than one word for a meaning (synonyms)?

2. Does the child misunderstand relations among words within utterances?

3. Does the child misunderstand words conveying the perspective of the speaker and other qualifying and descriptive terms of time, space, and amount?

4. Does the child consider semantic relations within utterances, attending to the interaction of semantic and syntactic relationships?

5. Does the child consider intersentence relationships?

6. Does the child include composite meanings of utterances in interpretation of the message?

7. Does the child include the influence of situation on the interpretation of meaning?

Receptive Deficiencies of Form   As discussed in the section on expression of language form, language *form* is the linguistic structure of utterances—articulation, pronunciation, word and sound sequencing, use of grammatical rules, structural complexity and adequacy, sentence types, and grammatical morphemes. Structural aspects of language supply information about the message. Difficulty in knowledge of linguistic structure interferes with interpretation of the complete message. For example, the interpretation of morphological and syntactical forms can affect understanding the information those forms carry. Rosenthal (1970) and Semel and Wiig (1975) observed that language-deficient children have difficulty understanding and interpreting utterances when the utterances increase in structural complexity and syntactic compression. For example, if the child does not fully understand the differences among prepositions, then the information conveyed by those prepositions, such as direction, location, and position, may not be understood by the child.

Adult	*Child*
Throw the ball *behind* the box.	Is that right? *(throws ball* in *the box)*

Understanding of the meaning signaled by bound morphemes may be missing in some children with language disorders. If a child does not understand verb differences of tense and plurality, the meaning of a sentence may be lost.

Adult	*Child*
The boys came over to play.	He did?

The process of embedding one clause within another may obscure meaning for a child with receptive problems, as might the differences between question forms and declarative utterances. Use of conjunctions may confuse a child who is unable to determine the differences signaled by "but" and "and" and "if. " The word "and" relates two ideas; "but" contrasts them; "if" presents a conditional state for consideration. A language-impaired child may not recognize the meaning signaled by the conjunctions.

Older Brother	*Language-Impaired Child*
You could go *if* I go, *but* I'm not going.	Good! I can go? You're not going?

Embedded clauses also interfere with complete understanding of an utterance by a language-impaired child, who may fail to recognize the relationship between the dominant and subordinate clauses.

Adult	*Child*
Mother said *that you can go.*	I can't go. Mother doesn't want me to.

Differences marked by word order may also not be identified by a language-
impaired child. Therefore, when a speaker says "John hit Jane," the child
may not be able to recognize who did the hitting or who got hit. This form
of error in reception seems to involve a combination of semantic and syntactic deficiencies.

Assessment of Receptive Language Form: Quantitative
Methods

Assessment of receptive abilities of structure should measure morphological rules, word sequences, and grammatical forms. Examples of
quantitative assessment tools of *form* include the following:

1. *Michigan Picture Language Inventory:* Language Structure subtest (Wolski,
   1962)
   Designed to evaluate word classes and function words. Designed to elicit oral
   responses; however, if the oral response to an item is incorrect, comprehension of grammatical structures can be assessed
2. *Assessment of Children's Language Comprehension:* (Foster, Gidden, and
   Stark, 1972)
   Primarily a measure of comprehension of sequence words; however, the
   introduction of the verbal elements in the vocabulary section includes items
   of syntax and morphology
3. *Northwestern Syntax Screening Test:* Receptive subtest (Lee, 1969)
   Measures comprehension of various syntactic structures (Spanish version
   available)
4. *Test for Auditory Comprehension of Language:* (Carrow, 1973)
   Assesses comprehension of items in four grammatical categories (Spanish
   version available)
5. *Test of Language Development:* Grammatic Understanding Subtest (Newcomer and Hammill, 1977)
   Determines a child's skills in processing certain syntactic structures
6. *Clinical Evaluation of Language Functions:* Processing Word and Sentence
   Structure Subtest (Semel and Wiig, 1980)
   Evaluates a child's ability to process and interpret utterance structures, including prepositional phrases, pronouns, verb phrases, modifiers, and negations

Assessment of Receptive Language Form: Qualitative
Methods

Assessment of receptive abilities of form in clinical observation may
include the following questions:

1. Does the child interpret information conveyed by prepositions?
2. Does the child understand verb differences expressed by tense and plurality?
3. Does the child recognize the signaling of meanings conveyed by conjunctions?
4. Does the child interpret the relationship between dominant and subordinate clauses?
5. Does the child recognize differences conveyed by word ordering?

This list is not intended to be exhaustive, but only to provide examples of formal assessment devices useful in evaluating a child's comprehension of speech. Other measures of intelligence offer measurement tools that yield information about a child's understanding of meaning (Terman and Merrill, 1969; Wechsler, 1949).

Assessing the reception of use, content, and form in language-disordered children is an important aspect of language evaluation, although adequate comprehension does not imply adequate production. The clinician must also recognize that a child's use of words does not imply that the child fully understands words and their application (Lucas, 1980).

Combinatorial Deficiencies The complex integrative nature of our language system makes it hard to imagine that a single, self-contained aspect of language learning can be impaired without affecting the other components of the system. Any child with a deficiency in language use, content, or form is a potential smorgasbord of disorders. It would be highly unusual for an assessment or intervention program to address isolated components of language without considering the entire system. Just as the range of language deficiencies varies from severe to mild, the combinations of impaired-language components are numerous. A child with comprehension problems is likely to have expressive deficiencies as well. For example, consider this parent's description of inadequate language:

> She cannot express herself. She is frustrated by new things and by not being able to do things perfectly the first time. She often does not grasp the meaning of things when you talk to her, and you have to tell her things in lots of different ways before she catches on.

Any number of combinations of language-learning deficits are possible. Some children with telegraphic speech may have general organizational problems. Others may do well if each sensory channel is evaluated in isolation from the others, but they may not be able to perform well if they must integrate what they hear with what they see, or if they must write the sounds they say. Children can fail in academic work without showing significant deficits on many standardized tests. A school diagnostician provided the following summary of testing on a second-grader who was failing:

There were no significantly low scores on the *Wechsler Intelligence Scale for Children (WISC)* and no scatter among the subtests. The discrepancy between verbal and performance-scaled scores was not significant. Conversational skills were adequate, and the *Bender Visual Motor Gestalt* score (Koppitz scale) was adequate for age level. Auditory discrimination scores as measured by paired word tests was adequate; memory and sound blending were good. These test results indicate that J. has no significant learning deficits that can account for his failure to read and perform in the classroom.

In later assessment it was noted that the child was fairly well coordinated but could not perform fine motor tasks, was a slow dresser and eater, and was rarely able to complete instructions at home or at school. The child could name a letter of the alphabet or any corresponding sound, but could not write it; he could read any written letter, but could not produce the corresponding sound. He obviously had some problems not identified with formal testing but which were interfering with his school achievement. Assessment must incorporate observations of the child's abilities outside formal testing in a variety of academic and social situations.

Written Language Disorders A language system and its use are not necessarily restricted to the spoken word. Written messages are used for communication and learning, just as are spoken messages. It is not unusual to find that deficiencies in oral language also appear in written language. An eloquent argument can be made for the position that once words are written they are no longer within the realm of one who studies normal and deficient language. Apparently it is this philosophy that has allowed some clinicians to approach reading disorders as if they were based solely on visual-perceptual problems.

Some children have severe visual-perceptual difficulties that are identified when written language disorders are discovered. Some authors conclude that reading disabilities result primarily from language deficits complicated by visual perception problems (Vellutino, 1979; Wiig and Semel, 1980). Other studies indicate that reading deficits are related to visual-verbal integration impairment and not to deficiencies in visual memory (Swanson, 1968).

The relationship between spoken sound and written symbol is fairly complex. English writing systems are based on sound-segmentation of the spoken language, and as Rees (1974) points out, humans cannot learn language if they are limited to some form of visual display of the language. Reading is the use of written symbols to translate one type of meaning symbols into another (Venezky, 1968; Vellutino, 1979). However, the transfer of spoken symbols to written symbols is not just the stringing together of sounds and letters in corresponding fashion (Liberman, 1973; Snyder, 1980; Wallach and Lee, 1980). The failure of language-deficient children to analyze what they hear and say frequently carries over into attempts to analyze what they read and write. Language-impaired readers often seem unaware of word components or sentence parts in either oral or written language (Snyder, 1980). They do not proofread for spelling or grammatical errors, cannot make reading or writing mistakes on purpose, and are unable to correct their own errors. Language-disordered children seldom interpret the implied message or comprehend the theme of a story even though they understand the words. They cannot interpret ambiguous written messages any better than they can interpret spoken ambiguities.

Some children's performances deteriorate dramatically when they must translate auditory information into motor activity, such as that required to match a sound to a printed letter or to write from dictation. It seems that the transfer of information from one sensory pathway to another is difficult. The basis of phonics and word-attack skills is the meaningful translation of sounds to letters to meaningful symbols. Children who do not learn to make the aural-to-visual transfer have difficulty learning to read.

Snyder (1980) reports that many poor readers have difficulty "forming equivalences" required in sound-letter matching. Rudel, Denckla, and Spalten (1976) compared poor readers with normal readers on their ability to associate Morse Code with letters, and to associate Braille type with letter names. The poor readers performed significantly worse than the normal readers, suggesting a problem in formation and recognition of equivalences (for instance, when symbols or components in one system are not recognized in another system). Liberman (1973) notes that the ability to analyze words into their constituent phonemes is a metalinguistic skill that children acquire between six and eight years of age. Analysis of written words requires that a child disassociate himself/herself from the word meaning and listen to the constituent sounds. This requires high-level knowledge of the sound system, which develops relatively late in normal children (Snyder, 1980). Many poor readers have difficulty analyzing the sound or letter elements of words, especially when auditory information is paired with visual equivalents.

The Problem and the Territory Language is the common component of reading and listening. Oral language deficits may affect other learning. Since reading includes oral language skills and knowledge of the native language, it is reasonable to assume that reading and writing skills are affected by oral language impairment. If a child cannot use syntactical knowledge to predict words, reading becomes a word-by-word or sound-by-sound effort. Syntactical knowledge helps the child determine the information in the reading material. Reading is a complex skill depending on many components of linguistic knowledge in response to graphic display (Snyder, 1980; Wiig and Semel, 1980). Snyder (1980, p. 35) points out that reading is not a "single-step translation of letter strings to their linguistic referents."

Roth and Perfetti (1980) suggest that reading comprehension depends on at least three kinds of information.

1. Syntactic structure and semantic properties of words in the sentence
2. Linguistic context
3. Reader's knowledge of the relationships referred to in the sentence

Poor readers seem to make less use of their knowledge of the world to comprehend stories (Smiley, Oakley, Worthen, Campione, and Brown, 1977). Some authors note that poor readers have difficulty understanding the relationship among ideas when they are in separate sentences and have less difficulty when the ideas are linked in single sentences (Marshall and Glock, 1978–79).

The pervasive influence of language on reading is obvious. Many language specialists consider written language deficiencies linguistic in nature (Vellutino, 1979; Rees, 1974). Mattingly (1972) suggests that the efficient reader must have two types of linguistic ability—primary linguistic activity and linguistic awareness. Primary linguistic activity, as described by Mattingly, is the ability to apply a set of internalized rules to the processing and production of language. Linguistic awareness enables children to reflect on language and analyze its components.

There is little scientific evidence that reading problems are based primarily on auditory or visual perceptual deficits (Rees, 1974), although historically the literature on reading disabilities and learning disorders has emphasized underlying perceptual motor deficits (Hallahan and Cruickshank, 1973). This theory has been challenged by those who consider reading a secondary language skill and relate reading disorders to linguistic deficits (Johnson and Myklebust, 1967; Calfee, Chapman, and Venezky, 1972; Klasen, 1972; Rees, 1974; Wiig and Semel, 1980). Evidently the beginning reader is more dependent on graphic information and deliberate decoding of the letters into their oral language equivalents (Snyder, 1980; Wiig and Semel, 1980). Advanced readers, however, handle visual decoding automatically, giving the syntactic and semantic components of the message greater attention. Children with reading problems may have extra difficulty because their attention is disrupted by poor coding skills and poor mnemonic devices (association clues) so that they do not retain what they read (Perfetti and Lesgold, 1977).

The relationship of oral language to written language is apparent. The language specialist should be responsible for the fundamentals of language necessary for transmitting oral language to written form and for helping the language-deficient child acquire linguistic awareness for written language (Rees, 1974). Assessment of written language should include analysis of the components of form, content, and use in both comprehension and expression, just as the assessment of oral language should.

Selective Attention It is difficult to identify all the factors influencing language development and to describe all those appearing in conjunction with language disorders. One aspect of functioning frequently associated with language disorders is that of memory and attention. Bloom and Lahey (1973) comment that the number of unrelated words a person must remember to learn a language is not determined, although children with poor language skills also frequently have poor memories for verbal information. The cause-and-effect relationship between memory for auditory information and language development is not established, although language-impaired children and adolescents have displayed memory deficits in the recall of numbers, names, or content (Wiig and Semel, 1980). However, it seems that an improvement in memory for auditory input may not influence language abilities and an improvement in language abilities may not affect scores on memory tests (Bloom, 1978). Deficits in remembering verbal information may be limitations of ability to store structural forms (Menyuk, 1969), or even problems with selective attention.

Language-disordered children generally have difficulty scanning and filtering unnecessary or misleading input. Inadequate filtering of information, such as being unable to focus on the message and rule out extraneous noise, makes it difficult for a child to determine which aspects of expression are necessary and important. For example, Hallahan, Gajar, Cohen, and Tarver (1978) studied 28 normal adolescent speakers and 20 language-impaired adolescents in an attempt to define some of the variables associated with learning competence and difficulty. A deficiency in selective attention differentiated the language-impaired children from the normal language speakers. The authors concluded that when children do not learn adequately from what they see and hear, one factor in their inadequate learning is improper attention to input.

Whatever the source of the constraints, the inability to receive and/or follow directions and attend to and recall sequences of events and details interferes with achievement in the language-disordered child. Some language-impaired children respond to instructions as if they had not retained their sequence; others have trouble remembering such rote sequences as the alphabet, phone numbers, or the multiplication tables. Difficulty remembering or paying attention seems to interfere with many facets of interaction and achievement (carrying out directions, remembering what the question is long enough to consider the answer, retaining sound or syllable sequencing). Many children who do not retain or attend to auditory information are proficient with visual and experiential information. They may recall in detail, for example, flying a kite with Uncle Ed two years ago, or the route to take to school, but they cannot recall what mother said to do before they could get an ice cream cone.

Some measures of language proficiency appear to be contaminated by memory requirements vital to completing a task. Directions often are complex, and the time between instructions and beginning the test items may be so long that the child forgets what the task is. The language-impaired child may not know to ask for reinstruction, or may not even declare that the instructions have been forgotten. When normal listeners miss an instruction or direction, they usually know that they've missed something.

Remediation is a problem-solving process for an ever-changing and complex problem. As the intervention continues, so must the assessment. The language skills that a child learns in clinical situations may not generalize into everyday living, so it is the responsibility of the clinician to determine what must be done to help the child transfer new skills into useful communication tools. The success of any language program rests on the child's acquiring communicative competence and experiencing the resultant rewards.

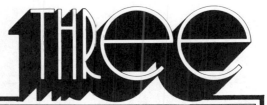

Intervention

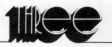

In normal language development, children are "... exposed to language in context ...," learn language in an "... active, creative process ...," and language is a "means-to-an-end ... for communication." (Johnson, 1976, p. 113). In light of this knowledge of normal language development, intervention should incorporate the philosophy that

1. Language does not exist apart from meaning
2. Children learn through active participation, not through passive imitation
3. Language serves as a tool for communication and learning, not as a final product

Efforts at improving communicative competence in language-deficient children should be directed toward the usefulness of language as a *vehicle for interaction* and a *device for learning and personal growth.*

Intervention has many components, including *direct intervention, indirect intervention,* and *use of resources and referrals.* Direct intervention integrates various diagnostic information, prognostic indications, and intervention techniques with content. Indirect intervention involves working with parents and teachers to help them understand the child's language deficiencies and guide them in constructive living and teaching situations with the child. The use of resources and referrals includes interacting with other agencies and professionals whose services also are necessary for the intervention program. Samples of these components of intervention are offered in this section and are intended only to be representative of some common patterns of intervention with school-age children and adolescents. Readers must consider the contents of each section in relation to the language-deficient people of their own experience.

○ DIRECT INTERVENTION

Intervention has to have a starting point, often before the evaluation process is completed, and sometimes in the face of numerous unanswered questions regarding the child's communication behaviors. Components of the formal intervention program must be identified, although the intervention process begins with the first suspicion of a language disorder and sometimes seems to have no end. As the suspected problems are identified and described in the evaluation process, the early plans of intervention materialize.

prioritizing the components of the intervention process

Beginning an intervention program never means that evaluation has ended, but intervening requires that priorities be established. Considerations in prioritizing the components of the intervention process include the following:

1. *Components of the communication disorder that seem most disruptive to communication (for example, no speech, no gesture system, limited comprehension, unintelligible speech).* The clinician must determine what is immediately critical for the child's communication needs and begin to alleviate whatever is interfering with meeting those needs.

2. *Communicative deficiencies that elicit the most negative reactions to the child.* Sometimes parents or teachers focus on minor features or by-products of the communication problem. While the minor features may not be the core of the disorder in the clinician's eyes, the perception of the child by people around him/her is important to the child's dynamic growth. The cosmetic aspects of communication breakdown need to be considered, as well as actual language form and function. For example, a protruding tongue does more to signal "dummy" to some teachers than a misused pronoun. Inability to follow directions in group work may interfere more in classroom activities than defective sentence construction. Some children develop odd mannerisms because they are aware of their failures. The mannerisms themselves can be annoying.

"Tommy, do *not* hit your head with your pencil every time you have to erase! It bothers people to see you do that!"

3. *Features of the communication disorder that are most distressing to the patient (if not already addressed in the above items).* Children become worried about themselves and sometimes focus on a particular symptom that they feel is a major problem. When possible, the clinician should find out what the child's worries are; comfort him/her with simple, direct information about his/her language learning deficiencies and personal strengths; and address some of his/her concerns in the intervention program

Clinician	Child
"What do you mean you think you're dumb?"	"I can't tell time, and everybody else can."

4. *Amount of time available for work with the patient, both within each session and long-term.* If the child is going to be in therapy for only a short period of time before moving to another school, clinician, or home, the clinician must consider what will create the most effective changes in that time period. Some

aspects of communication deficiencies lend themselves to change in limited time spans; others require long-term, intensive work. Some children can work only a few minutes at a time before they lose concentration or willingness to participate. Their sessions must be short and end before they reach that point.

The focus on intervention with language-deficient children is on maximizing communication effectiveness. The various components of language deficiencies should not be treated as unrelated wounds to be medicated or defective parts to be replaced, but rather as interdependent symptoms of an inadequately functioning language system. One reason behind the search for linguistic universals is the need for assistance in determining a reasonable course of intervention with the language-impaired population. We continue trying to identify levels at which all children proceed systematically in their language acquisition so that we can intervene appropriately when normal acquisition fails. Clinicians are tantalized by developmental norms when planning intervention programs but sometimes find the use of normative information alone inadequate for designing approaches to intervention and for predicting success of intervention. Other bases for prognosis need to be considered.

predicting the success of intervention

Intervention requires that the clinician consider the communicative future of the child; that is, given ideal evaluation, intervention, and change, what can be predicted about the child's potential communicative functioning? Usually, long-term predictions, such as the one posed by the preceding question, are only for the clinician's private consideration and may change as the clinician learns more about the child. Projections should be based on all available data regarding the child's communicative functioning and should be used wisely to gauge intervention plans. The data on which the clinician bases judgments about the child should include more than test scores and may include:

1. Rate of learning over time
2. Number of subsystems included
3. Attention span
4. Motivation of the child and level of awareness about the problem
5. Supportiveness of environment (availability of others to reinforce new learning)

Although test data and language analyses are of value to the clinician in making predictions about a child's communicative future, they should be considered within the context of clinician-child interaction. An experienced and competent clinician can cultivate a clinical impression of the child as they participate together in the evaluation and intervention experiences. Many creative and successful interventions have occurred because an insightful clinician trusted a hunch about a child or his/her potential.

change in intervention

Change in child language can be a disconcerting aspect of remediation, as well as a relief. Many clinicians become distressed as they try to determine what to "do next." A change in child language may lead to more difficult intervention problems than the original pattern of symptoms in the sense that therapeutic and communication complexities increase as language-skills increase. In some ways, for example, it is easier to work with a nonverbal child in teaching language precursors and early word meaning than it is to change telegraphic speech into well-organized and complete utterances. It is simpler, in many instances, to present two-part and three-part semantic relations to a child than it is to help a child learn the construction and function of embedded sentences. Change appears in various forms, and the clinician may find its presence harder to manage than its absence. Some basic components of flexibility in the intervention process include observing change in the child as well as adaptations the clinician must make. For example:

1. Analyzing changes in the child's language structure, content, use, and style throughout the course of intervention
2. Using the child's experiences, body, reactions, and interests as gauges of change, versus using prescriptive programs or teaching sequences from predesigned teaching packages
3. Detecting errors in the intervention plans or hypotheses that form the bases of intervention and contemplating changes in the plans (for example, direct intervention, tutoring, changing structure within the child's life, changing emphasis of work within the intervention activities)

Ongoing evaluation as a part of intervention does not imply that changes must be made at every hesitation in the intervention program. The remediation specialist often needs to keep on trying in the face of no obvious change. Clinicians need to be cautious about changing intervention goals or strategies prematurely. The remediation specialist occasionally falls into the premature-change trap, because temporary plateaus in improvement are reached, or because the child's responses are not tested in real situations. Some real-life testing of the new behaviors can keep the clinician from jumping to conclusions about a child's communicative competencies. If the child does not use new language skills with increasing frequency and in a variety of communication settings, the clinician cannot assume that the material is within the child's control and part of the communication repertoire.

It is important to consider the differences between the thoughtful intervention of a trained professional and the automated work of a technician.
Prescriptive services are in vogue in many public and private work settings,
and the intervention specialist may be employed in a consultative role to
evaluate children's language and to write language programs for someone
else to execute. Some knowledgeable writers speak of the speech-language
specialist as one who enters into "prescriptive teaching" (Yassi, 1978). The
clinician should exercise caution when considering prescriptive consultation. Prescriptive evaluation usually means that the clinician sees a child two
or three times for assessment and then writes a program of intervention for
someone else to carry out. This removes the important ongoing aspects of
evaluation as part of the intervention program and constant change as part
of that evaluation. One of the greatest values of successful intervention is
the dynamic interaction between child and clinician in which the clinician
responds to the child and the child's language; intervention can then be
adapted to the child's needs and what he/she brings to each session.

As a language learner the child must be a partner in communicative
interaction. Language acquisition includes . . . "early interactive experiences in which the child acts as participant rather than as object or observer"
(Rees, 1978, p. 233). Children learn language in context, and communicative interaction is the source and context of language learning. Bowerman
(1978) notes that children are not passive language learners; they exhibit
highly effective methods of learning when they can control verbal interactions. In many clinical settings, the pattern of interaction is arranged so that
the language-impaired child is directed to perform in a certain way, regardless of his/her interest or needs at the time (Grossfield & Geller, 1980).
According to Bowerman (1978) this is the kind of interaction least conducive to language development.

intervention approaches

Various assessment procedures and studies of child language disabilities have led to the conclusion that language impairment represents
language delay and not language disorder (Leonard, 1972; Morehead and
Ingram, 1973; Wiig and Semel, 1976). That is, language-impaired children
show delayed but developmentally sequenced language abilities. This is in
contrast to the theory that some language-impaired children exhibit irregular language learning not developmentally comparable to younger, normal-
speaking children (Berry, 1969; Menyuk, 1969). Although this argument is
not examined in this discussion, the implications of the developmental
model for remediation approaches should be considered.

Developmental hierarchies should form the basis of intervention so that language behaviors can be assigned a developmental equivalent and then
coached into increasingly more difficult levels of functioning.

Analysis of the child's language disorder should be the basis of intervention
so that deficiencies can be charted and remediation can be based on modifying the child's deficiencies.

A developmental approach takes the logical stand that the best place to
begin a language intervention program is with the simplest or smallest
language unit, advancing from there. This premise is based on the assumption that normal language learners begin language acquisition at the simplest level and progress through the most complex phases in an orderly
fashion. Wiig and Semel (1976; 1980) state that remedial procedures should
reflect developmental sequences, or order of difficulty, as indicated by clinical observations and/or research. This logic is difficult to apply because in
many instances we do not know what constitutes the smallest unit of language, nor how advances in normal language change are made. Our assumptions about simplicity may be wrong, and what seem to be the simplest
structures or functions may not really be. Developmental milestones and
ordinal hierarchies offer certain kinds of developmental checkpoints, but
across categories language "seems too complex to be captured by a developmental progression" (Siegel and Spradlin, 1978, p. 370). For example,
in teaching word combinations we may teach a core vocabulary and then
encourage a child to combine the words. However, reducing sentences to
single words in which communicative intent is omitted may increase the
difficulty, not decrease it (Muma, 1978). Attempts to simplify the language
task may make it more difficult.

Contrasting a remedial approach to intervention with a developmental
approach points up the fact that a remedial approach requires the clinician
to analyze the language disorder by describing deficiencies in observable
behaviors and to base intervention on deficient characteristics. Remedial
approaches do not always provide the clinician with the necessary help for
working with older language-deficient children. The complexities of their
language dysfunctions defy attempts to describe their language behaviors,
making it difficult to determine which deficiencies are the best targets for
intervention.

Embracing any single intervention approach to the exclusion of all others
means embracing the deficits of the approach as well as the assets. The
ultimate responsibility of the language clinician is to determine what is
important for the child and how the child can change ineffective language
efforts into successful communication activities. The clinician must analyze
the components of normal language and apply that knowledge to understanding deficiencies in each child's language. It seems that a combined use

of both developmental and remedial approaches offers the greatest benefit for clinicians who attempt to intervene with school-age language-deficient children. No intervention approach, strategy, or technique is likely to be successful in isolation from the others because intervention requirements change as the child changes, and each clinician must select the best strategy for the situation.

Teaching Techniques and Strategies It is imperative that intervention supply the means for children to learn the application of in-session language skills to daily communication experiences. The basis of intervention lies in acknowledgement that the primary functions of language are for communication and for learning, and that learning a language is a process and not a product. With this commonsense approach to intervention, it is a marvel that it has taken some of us so long to stop depending totally on sentence frames and imitation drills to change deficient communication.

Imitation

Imitation, as one technique in the clinician's teaching repertoire, is not to be disregarded totally. It seems relevant to remediation programs for language-deficient children in at least two ways.

> Direct reinforced imitative training may enhance the precision of a child's responses as he/she attempts closer approximations of adult speech.
>
> Verbal imitation may be a predictor of subsequent linguistic development in some language impaired-children (Siegel and Spradlin, 1978).

Imitative training in its richest form can include the possibility for learning meaning within context. Presenting a verbal stimulus alone in imitation training may interfere with subsequent language acquisition if the child is not directed to apply the linguistic form in nonimitative contexts. Any technique must help the child transfer newly learned aspects of language to communicative interactions.

Rules and Drills

Intervention programs that drill children in sets of rule-based behaviors are not adequate unless the intervention includes helping the child learn to apply the rules in communication. Trantham and Pedersen (1976) discuss drill-based learning in a creative, communicative context, which is different from a prepared language program that encourages rote learning. Their drills for grammatical rule learning are immediately transferred to interactive situations; children then learn to apply and monitor their use of the grammatical forms, emphasizing meaningful use of new language forms.

Reinforcement

Behavior modification approaches to language teaching traditionally define the components of language at the morpheme/syntax level and at the phoneme level. They describe basic concepts in behavior modification terms (operant learning, imitative learning, prompting, target behaviors, response rate, reward contingencies, and so on) (Miller and Yoder, 1972). The application of behavioral models often incorporates verbal imitation, as seen in some articulation programs, stuttering controls, and sentence pattern drills.

Ruder (1978) discusses behavior management and reinforcers in the training sequence, which includes attention to language use as well as form. He notes that for every language structure to be trained, an underlying use should be delineated. According to Ruder, in carry-over programming that he has implemented, target behaviors and training steps are part of teaching the child to use linguistic rules in everyday situations.

It is difficult to apply behavior modification principles directly to conversational discourse because of the number and complexity of variables in communicative interaction. In my clinical experience, the rigid application of behavior modification principles has not been helpful in teaching children to bridge the gap between linguistic performance and communicative competence. I have taught numbers of children to parrot phrases and use them in certain situations without teaching them to attend to the communicative use of their utterances. They can talk, but they don't know why or when.

Programming and reinforcing a series of isolated language behaviors do not seem to have a maximally positive effect in changing children's communication. de Villiers and de Villiers (1978) note that children are more likely to get their meaning across if they speak correctly and more likely to be misinterpreted if they speak inadequately, concluding that the most effective reinforcer is successful communication. The language-deficient child needs to learn to profit from the communication success of language use; clinicians must devise ways of encouraging language-deficient children to judge the accuracy of their own understanding of speech, to notice if their listeners understand them, and to attempt to change the way they convey their messages if they are not interpreted correctly. As Muma (1978) points out, behavior modification may be effective in altering performance, but there is some question regarding its effect on communicative competence.

Teaching Materials and Programs

Many clinicians have access to predesigned teaching programs and packages. Because their goals and teaching sequences may be stated simply, one can easily justify their use. A teaching program is a device to be put at the service of a competent clinician, who, in turn, is at the service of the language-deficient patient. Any program should be a tool that the clinician uses in discovering systematic and creative ways of working with language deficiencies in children.

Teaching materials and packages may contribute to intervention by helping to describe aspects of language behavior. As Siegel and Spradlin (1978) note, prepared programs often suggest sequences of presentation and clinical options regarding content. A good program is not designed to replace a thinking clinician but can aid a knowledgeable specialist when the program is applied in ways that build on the principles incorporated in the program and are applicable to the language deviations of each child.

Group and Individual Intervention

Another option for intervention is group therapy. Matching children for group therapy should be done carefully and with the purpose of enhancing, not diluting, the therapeutic experience. In certain instances individual therapy is indicated; for example, when behavior or rate of progress in one child can hinder the improvement of another child. However, when scheduling permits, matching children who have related therapeutic needs, who have similar predicted rates of improvement, and who are behaviorally compatible, can produce greater therapeutic benefits than isolating each child for intervention. With groups of two, three, or four, the clinician can enhance learning of group members by setting up situations in which the children learn to do the following:

1. Interact with each other using their present levels of language skill
2. Listen to and understand less-than-perfect speakers and read and comprehend less-than-perfect writers
3. Monitor the spoken or written work of another person, and learn to declare that they have failed to understand the message
4. Apply newly learned language skills in supervised interactions
5. Correct the mistakes of another speaker/writer
6. Support others in the course of correction and errors during intervention

A well-constructed group can reassure a child that he/she is not the only person needing intervention. Older children often need affirmation of their strengths, and a group of peers is a good place to find support. They can be apprised of their communication deficits in a supportive way and praised for their accomplishments in full view of group members. Group sharing of problems in deficits can lead to constructive changes that a therapist alone could not achieve. For example:

Child A	Child B
I got another F in English	Why?
I forgot to do my homework	Oh, yeah, I have to write my assignments down in a calendar. If I don't I always forget.
Huh! Maybe *I'll* get a calendar too.	

remediation of expressive deficiencies

The process of intervention represents intense communicative interaction. It should be designed to take into account the relationships among linguistic structures, contents, and the uses to which language is put. Intervention suggestions in this section are only examples of the various approaches that remediation *can* take. They present selected areas of intervention with language deficiencies of use, content, or form. Examples represent a composite of personal clinical experience, as well as implications from and adaptations of current literature. An important point to note is that intervention identified for one component includes dimensions of other components of the language system. For example, remediation of expressive deficiences of *use* encompasses aspects of *content* and *form;* remediation of expressive deficiencies of *form* includes *use* and *content.* When one uses language to teach language, it is not always desirable or possible to separate components of the language system.

Remediation of Expressive Language Use A variety of contextual and environmental factors influences a child's knowledge of utterance use. Development of adequate production skills includes learning to convey meaning with spoken or written symbols, as well as with appropriate situational elements that help convey the message and its intent. As the desired effect of the communication occurs, or does not occur, the normal child learns that messages are not always received as they were intended (Rees, 1978). Language-impaired people do not always learn this lesson, nor how to revise their messages to repair a communication breakdown.

Communicating with Others

Every remediation session should include conversation and interaction, so that the language-deficient child can respond to a listener in a controlled situation and learn to change his/her utterances as a result of the listener's response. The clinician can ask leading questions or pretend to misunderstand the child's intent to show him/her what aspects of the intended communication caused the communication breakdown. In those situations the child can be guided toward changing the message (Wallach and Lee, 1980). Intervention should also include some time for the lan-guage-impaired child to interact with other children (Fey, Leonard, and Wilcox, 1981). The clinician then has an opportunity to observe the child's language use, content, and form, in real-life situations, and the language-impaired child has an opportunity to use new language skills. Another child may not know the intended message nor how to ask for additional informa-tion; a linguistically superior child may instruct the language-impaired child in how to supply necessary information. Fey, Leonard, and Wilcox (1981) suggest that the language-impaired child should have the chance to interact with children of similar or poorer language skills. They observe that these situations place fewer constraints on the language-impaired child in conver-sational participation and may provide the child with the opportunity to become a more active communicator by practicing newly learned language skills in a nonthreatening situation. Careful monitoring of these conversa-tional situations gives the clinician many opportunities to point out to the language-impaired child what information is needed, how the message was missent or misinterpreted by the listener. In some situations, the language-deficient child can learn how to instruct another child in conversational requirements.

An intervention strategy using conversation as a device for learning and applying language should not be confused with free time or unguided play time. The observed interaction between language-impaired children and other children can provide the clinician with valuable teaching opportuni-ties. Intervention designs that include planned interaction as part of inter-vention might include the following:

1. *Conveying intended messages* This requires choosing the best word combi-nations, understanding the combination of verbal and nonverbal information given by the conversation partner, and monitoring the listener's under-standing of the message. The following are examples illustrating ways in which a child can learn to monitor the effectiveness of his/her utterances:

    a. by directing and correcting the work of other children. The child must determine if his/her companions responded to the instructions and if they performed in the intended way. These experiences should include oppor-tunities to learn to change the way the message is expressed if the other child does not receive the intended message.

    b. by directing the clinician with certain messages, monitoring the clinician's responses, and altering directions when needed. This might include allow-ing the child to be the "teacher," who must monitor and correct.

"Here's a car, Bobby.

Here's a box. You're the teacher. Tell me something to do with the box or the car."

The clinician then reacts literally to the child's instructions, calling the child's attention to how the actions were the result of misconveyed messages. The clinician can then suggest alternate ways for the child to try to obtain the desired results. This suggestion is particularly adaptable to children who do not indicate semantic propositions with such markers as prepositions. For example, "Put it the box" will not bring any results but a complaint from the clinician that the instruction is unclear. The clinician can prompt the child, "Do you mean *on* or *in* the box?" The child must then be asked to judge the clinician's accuracy of response in light of the child's own instructions.

2. *Staying on the topic* This task includes determining what the topic is and monitoring the content of verbal interchanges. For example:

   direct comments to the child—"That's not what we're talking about. We're talking about swimming and playing in water."

   redirecting the child's comments—"Wait a minute to tell us about your hurt knee. We're talking about swimming. You tell us one thing you like to do when you're *swimming*."

   asking the children in a group what they're "talking about"—such as discussing the fact that talking about a cut knee is not the same as "talking about" ice cream flavors.

   appointing someone in the group to name a topic for discussion, then assigning that person to monitor the discussion for the topic.

3. *Avoiding fillers and nonfunctional words that cloud the message.* The child may need direct instructions for conveying a clear message to the listener.

Clinician	*Child*
	My, uh, we, um, said, said, uh, my mother, got . . . I have. uh, she got yesterday, uh, she, you know, uh. before supper, you know, we, I mean, her hand, you know, on the stove and it hurt.
What did your mother do? My mother . . .	My mother burned her hand.
How did she burn it? Say, "on the_____	On the stove
When? Say, "yesterday, before_____	Yesterday before supper

4. *Learning the indirect use of words to convey nuances of communication and shades of interpersonal contact*
   Would you go?
   Could you get that?
   You *might* want to come over here.

5. *Changing meaning with facial expression, body movement, and intonation*
   a. A head shake, a laugh, or a wink may signal that the speaker intends a nonliteral meaning of what he/she said.
   b. Pointing to an object may change the topic of conversation suddenly with no verbal clue that the topic has changed.

6. *Learning to enhance information given to another person who has different perspectives of time, space, or direction, or who has not shared the same experiences as the speaker*
   a. using role playing to act out how people talk when they experience various emotions; adlibbing lines in a make-believe play (playing store, school, and others); acting out the characters in a story the clinician reads or the children write
   b. using body language and facial expression to illustrate how people look when they experience various emotions; having nonverbal conversations that show emotions, give directions, and ask questions using body movement and facial expressions only
   c. giving instructions or information in which no gestures are allowed and no questions permitted so that the child must change the verbal instructions until the listener responds appropriately

7. *Learning to determine the theme or point of a story or conversation by drawing together all the elements influencing the message and intent*
   a. giving titles to stories, or having the child relate an event and see if he/she can conclude one "lesson" or main idea from it
   b. contrasting the difference between telling the sequence of events and telling "what happened" in summary form
   c. having the child summarize long stories in one or two sentences
   d. trying to get the child to consider the reason for certain dialogues

Clinician	*Child*
"You just saw Tom come in to tell me someone cut his finger out in the hall. "Why do you think he told me that?"	"He wanted you to know."-or- "I don't know."

(Note: Once again, never assume the point is so obvious to the child that he/she is being flippant. My experience suggests that the child may adopt the literal interpretation because that really represents what he/she understands.)

Clinician	*Child*
"If he cut his finger, he's probably bleeding, and he may need help to fix it. Tom may think I can help.	I guess he wants you to fix it."
Now see if you can tell me why Tom told me about the person who cut himself?"	

It is difficult on such occasions to let the child outside continue to bleed and to control the pitch of your own voice, while trying to resolve a problem in reasoning with a language-deficient child; but, real situations often provide the best teaching opportunities.

A subtle trap for clinicians, as well as for parents, is the tendency to credit the child with "what he meant" (that is, responding to the intended message rather than the surface structure of the utterance). That stance is usually appropriate for relatives, but someone who wants to change language behaviors must indicate to the child that he/she has not fulfilled his/her part in conveying the message, and the listener cannot bear all the burden for both. As children get older, they must learn their responsibilities as speakers, as well as listeners, and be able to judge the effectiveness of their utterances. Language-deficient children frequently do not notice the quality of their speech or writing relative to their audience's informational needs and fail to provide adequate information for the interaction.

Interactive Styles and Codes

The limitations of language deficiencies sometimes lead language-deficient children to act in a way often considered distasteful, unpleasant, or odd. If systematic suggestions for behavior changes are not introduced as part of intervention, many children will never recognize why people around them respond to them negatively. Suggestions for change must be presented to the language impaired-child or adolescent in such a way that he/she is not left feeling criticized as a person. It is easy to imply that the child is a "bad" person when evaluating the child's public/social actions.

"Your voice is hurting my ears!"

"Quit talking to yourself like that."

' Why don't you pay attention to how I feel?"

"Quit acting like a goose and act right!"

Clinicians and parents need to be certain they are not feeling angry when they give advice about changing social behaviors. It is important that intervention regarding these matters reflect clinician insight and not personal annoyances. Areas where the clinician can intervene might include:

1. general appearance
(staring, talking to themselves, laughing for no apparent reason, scratching)

2. physical range of movements and use of space (too close or too distant for the interaction, overindulgence in physical contact, acting repulsed when another person reaches to touch)

3. use of a code appropriate to the listener, message, and situation (appropriateness of voice and content, respect for authority, awareness of sharing/giving with another)

4. social mores and mannerisms
(sex-appropriate behaviors, table manners, bodily functions, and interpretation of approval/disapproval through the nonverbal reactions of others)

Language specialists and teachers can expand these categories and add several of their own. All aspects of communicative style cannot be changed at once, but if style is considered important to communicative interactions then intervention must deal with deficient interactive style.

Use of Language to Analyze Language: Metalinguistic Behavior

Requiring children to monitor and manipulate language often requires judgments about language, or metalinguistic skills (Wallach and Lee, 1980). Intervention requires the child to consider and modify aspects of language. For example, asking a child to rhyme words, count words, segment syllables and sounds, and so forth requires knowledge *about* the structure of language (Snyder, 1980; Wallach & Lee, 1980). With limited instruction, normal school-age children can look at language *per se* with their own language, and learn to *talk about* words, sounds, and meanings. Language-impaired children are usually unable to monitor and correct their errors and frequently do not transfer the lessons from drill and rote work to communication situations.

The following suggestions represent possible intervention targets with children who are limited in their use of language to analyze language:

1. Identify words, sentences, and phrases that are possible English combinations, as well as those that are meaningful combinations.
   a. "Sometimes I . . ." Does that make sense?
   b. "Tag" Is that a word?

2. Correct semantic and syntactic errors in other's and the child's own utterances.
   a. grammar and word order
   b. omissions of words or word endings
   c. letter, word, sentence, and event sequencing in utterances
   d. punctuation

3. Make purposeful mistakes in a designated semantic or syntactic category such as those listed in item 2 above. Have a peer listen critically or proofread an utterance and then make corrections.
   You *said:* "We *was* going."
   You have to *say:* "We *were* going."

4. Rearrange misordered phrases, sentences, or word parts, discussing how word order changes meaning
   He is couching on the sleep.
   This is a girl happy.

5. Have the children teach peers or younger children tasks. Instructing another child in a task and correcting errors require analysis of another's work and attention to linguistic detail, and makes the child *talk about* elements of language.

6. Discuss *words* that can be *used* and *sentences* that can be *changed*.
   "My_____hat is gone." (*Name* five *words* I could use there.)
   "I_____in the lake." (Can I *use* an action *word?* Name five action words that would fit.)

"He will go to the door." (Make that into a *question.*)
"Can she come to my house?" (Make that into a *sentence that tells something.*)

7. Analyze written language with oral language.
   "Write a sentence. Read it and read exactly what you wrote, not what you think you wrote."

8. Analyze oral language with written language.
   "*Say* a sentence. *Write* what you said exactly as you said it. Is that *what you said?* Close your eyes and say it. Read *what you wrote.*"

   The importance of helping language-deficient children improve their use of language requires that we use language as a viable intervention target. Previous examples have discussed some ways of using dialogue as an instructive device. Whatever the objectives, language-deficient children must learn ways of conveying their intended messages and clarifying their utterances if the listener does not interpret it correctly. A legitimate aspect of intervention is showing children how their messages are unclear and showing them ways to change these messages. Such activities are compatible with the philosophy that intervention should try to make language more useful in meeting communication needs.

   Remediation of Expressive Language Content   School-age children who are unable to express content adequately present a wide variety of disorders: word choice and meaning, word retrieval and fluency, word combinations (semantic relations), and appropriate elaboration. Examples of these disorders are discussed in terms of possible intervention

1. *Word choice and meaning* Language-impaired children retain narrow meanings of words and often must rely on the context of the message to carry the meaning of separate words. Wiig and Semel (1980) suggest that intervention with word meaning deficits includes a wide variety of semantic and experiential contexts and teaching new words should range from the familiar and expected to the unfamiliar and unpredictable. Lucas (1980) notes that many language-impaired children make errors in word use related to time, space, and quality and quantity and offers specific suggestions for intervention with those errors.
   a. in some instances, a child's use of word meanings can be facilitated by teaching him/her how to define words. The quality and elaboration of the definition can also be used to gauge the child's understanding of the complexities of words
   b. refinement of classes of attributes (small-big, long-short, tall-thin, short-wide) is often helpful to language-impaired children. Beginning with the use of global terms (big-small), then specifying dimensions of subunits (length, depth, width, height) can demonstrate the variations and complexities of the words. Often it is beneficial to explain and illustrate the uses of the words and then have the child apply them in various situations. As the child becomes proficient with constant referents (to the height of the doors,

or the length of the table in the workroom) change the point of reference so that something once considered "big" is no longer big in relation to another object.

c. in some cases, the same word can apply to a different attribute of experience (for example, changing from distance to time referents with the word "long"). The child may need physical referents as the dimensions change relative to position, time, and space (long rope, long road, long trip, long talk, long time, long life). Another way of teaching the child to refine categories of referents is to specify differentiations within categories (variations of time, such as soon, not long, near, almost, about, next; variations of distance and proximity such as near, close, far away). Many children need explanations regarding the use of identical words referring to different dimensions (close to my house/close to my birthday).

2. *Word retrieval and fluency* Retrieval of the right word for communicative situations is generally difficult for the language-impaired child and intervention must focus on improving retrieval. It could include strategies for helping the child associate phonological or relational cues (words beginning with *s*, rhyming words), drills for rapid naming of labels or categorical items, and practicing sentence completion tasks (synonyms, antonyms) (Lucas, 1980; Wiig And Semel, 1980).

3. *Word combinations (semantic relations)* Errors in syntax or word order usually represent a basic problem in encoding semantic relations (Lucas, 1980). Some language-impaired children seem to defy rules for combining words, with such utterances as the *rain is clouding,* or *beans eat boys.* Sometimes it is possible to design intervention programs so that word combinations are built onto semantically simple utterances that increase systematically in complexity as the child's skills increase.

Semantic Role Combinations	*Example*
Actor + Action	John hits.
Action + Object	Hit the ball.
Actor + Action + Object	John hits the ball.
Action + Modified Object	Hit the big ball.
Actor + Action + Modified Object	John hits the big ball.
Modified Actor + Action + Modified Object	Baby John hits the big ball.

Additional intervention suggestions with word combinations that use words to project the situation, make inferences, and maintain the topic, include the following:

1. Using verbal analogies, problem-solving skills, and logic
2. Rearranging scrambled words and sentences
3. Completing stories and sentences with appropriate content

4. Employing cause-and-effect situations, emphasizing causality and similarity among objects or events

5. Using prior information to determine and express the whole idea of several sentences

6. Drawing conclusions from a series of pieces of information

It is so rare for a language-impaired child to produce language without criticism or correction that often intervention itself inhibits the learning of appropriate fluency and elaboration. Intervention may need to include time for the child to learn to elaborate a topic, describe feelings, brainstorm for new ideas, and practice the rapid expression of related topics.

The stilted drill of many therapeutic endeavors may impair rather than facilitate appropriate fluency of expression. General remediation suggestions with children who have content deficiencies include the following:

1. Do not rely on drill, utterance frames for imitation, or rote work as the primary intervention techniques. Encourage the child to vary his/her utterances to express the same meaning in various linguistic forms.

2. Make it obvious that the child's message is not clear when he/she does not provide enough information or words to convey the message. Tell the child what is needed and ask leading questions, to teach him/her how to supply the words the listener needs for understanding.

3. Emphasize at every opportunity that the child's speech must be meaningful for the listener and functional for the child. Do not assume that the child understands the meaning of the words that he/she uses or the implications of the utterances. Teach language-deficient children not to assume that just because they've said something they have conveyed their message. They need to know that words used *alone* are very different in meaning from the *same words used in combination* with other words.

4. Show the child that he/she can exercise some control over the environment and his/her interactions by choosing appropriate words. Change the task or the listeners, and have the child select the most appropriate words for the situation. (See the section on language *use.*)

The focus of intervention with children who have content disorders should not concentrate on word meanings alone, but should include application of the words for communicative interaction. An intervention program with content improvement as its primary goal is self-limiting and contrary to what we know about normal language acquisition and use. The content of an utterance is its meaning with respect to what the child is making language do for him/her (Halliday, 1973).

With the emphasis on accountability in many rehabilitation settings, clinicians have been hesitant to include conversation in their lesson plans because of the difficulty in defending such activities as legitimate. Many of my colleagues were trained not to "play games" in their intervention sessions, and to consider any strategy a waste of time if it did not produce behaviors that could be counted and tallied. The short-term objectives suggested in Samples 1 and 2 are based on Simon's suggested ways of writing lesson plans for children with communication disorders (Simon, 1979). They should prove helpful to the clinician considering ways to incorporate interactive language teaching into the language intervention program.

Sample 1: Expressive Disorder of Content and Use—
Short-Term Objectives

These behavioral objectives are designed to be used with a language-deficient child who exhibits inadequate verbal organization, one who has difficulty relating order of events, cannot support a point of view, and uses distracting speech fillers while not providing enough information.

1. The child will say at least 3 things to describe each of 25 pictures. He/she will rehearse subvocally before saying anything so that he/she can organize his/her output to allow no more than 20 percent of his/her utterances to include fillers.
2. The child will organize pictures sequentially into a logical story after having been told the story by the clinician. Using at least 10 unfamiliar sequence stories, he/she will appropriately describe each picture in the series and then state what the entire story was "about."
3. When asked by the clinician to state his/her opinion, the child will express 3 feelings or opinions about each of 25 pictures ("I like it." "I think it's dumb." "It's pretty to me.").
4. When asked by the clinician to state 3 facts about each of 25 pictures, the child will state observable or functional information ("It is red." "You can ride on it." "This kind holds more than a smaller one, because it has more room inside.").

Sample 2: Expressive Disorder of Content and Use—
Short term objectives

These behavioral objectives are applicable to language-deficient children whose language deficiencies include not asking questions to get needed information, not clarifying messages upon listener request, not listening for errors in their own speech, and not reading for errors in their written work.

1. In eight out of ten instances, the child will ask enough questions to complete a task assigned by the clinician when incomplete information has been given to him/her.

Clinician	Child
I want you to go stand by the _____.	Stand by what?
I want you to give me a certain color crayon.	What color?

2. In eight out of ten instances, the child will describe unfamiliar pictures to the clinician—with the clinician asking leading questions—to give him/her sufficient information to determine what the described item is.

Child	Clinician
I have something, and you eat it.	What category of food does it belong in?
It's a dessert and, you eat it after a meal.	How is it fixed, and what does it look like?
You put it in the refrigerator, and it looks all jiggly and red.	It must be jello.

3. The child will detect an error in the clinician's sentence constructions (pronoun, verb tense, noun-verb agreement, nonsense word for the sentence, or ommision of a word) eight out of ten times by restating the utterance correctly and naming which word had to be changed.

Clinician	Child
I am to town.	I am going to town. You left out *going*.

4. The child will detect written errors in simple sentences (word reversals in short sentences, word omissions, transposition of letters or word endings). For example, "I went *ot* town."

It should be noted that these very brief examples of short term objectives do not address the important aspect of carryover. A crucial measure of carryover for a new communicative behavior is its appearance in communicative interaction.

Remediation of Expressive Language Form   Errors in expressive language structure have been a popular target for intervention because of their observability and the easy identification of goals for change. However, many clinicians and parents have been frustrated with the slow or inadequate transfer of new structures to spontaneous speech, in spite of intensive drill on the new forms. It seems difficult to bridge the gap between linguistic structures in drill and linguistic structures in communication. One of the tasks of intervention is to bridge that gap.

Many aspects of linguistic structure could be used as examples of intervention strategies. Morpheme errors have been selected as one example of structural deficits often requiring intervention. Morpheme errors are affected by meaning, redundancy, and differentiation of their subclasses. Slobin (1971) and Brown (1973) suggested that children first learn forms that carry heavy phonetic load, stress, and prosodic features. Therefore, it appears that the teaching of forms in elliptical utterances where they occur alone and not within the context of other words will increase the acoustic load on the morpheme by adding phonetic stress ("Whose is that?" "Tom's.") Morphemes are acquired also on the basis of the meaning they convey (Slobin, 1971; Brown, 1973), and the less information they convey, or the more redundant the information is to the context, the more difficult they are to acquire. In elliptical forms, morphemes are not redundant as they are in full form (Brown 1973). The morpheme that stands alone (that is, uncontracted and unbound morphemes such as pronouns, prepositions, articles) seems to carry more phonetic load than bound morphemes (such as third person inflections: "he walks").

Information about the semantic and acoustic influence on morpheme acquisition in child language can be readily used in remediation tasks. Considerations for choosing morphemes for early emphasis in intervention are summarized as follows:

1. Unbound morphemes usually are easier to learn than bound morphemes (for example, a preposition should be easier to acquire than a plural inflection, "boys").
2. The semantic information the morpheme carries for the message should affect the ease of learning (for instance, preposition "in" conveys more information than the article "the").
3. The acoustic stress of the morpheme may influence learning (as an example, the morpheme in the elliptical utterance "Tom's" receives more stress than the morpheme embedded in an utterance "Tom's hat").

If a child conveys meaning with high content words but fails to use appropriate structural forms, he/she can learn the syntactic and morphological rules in structures where they carry the most meaning.

1. Emphasize the meaning of a morpheme by teaching a structure without the aid of words that make the morpheme redundant.

   Clinician shows picture of one cat
   We see the cat.
   Show me the cat.
   We see the ___.

Clinician shows picture of several cats

We see the cats.
Show me the cats.
We see the _____.

Clinician alternates picture of one cat with picture of several cats

We see the cat. (showing appropriate picture)
We see the cats. (showing appropriate picture)
Look at this picture.
It is a picture of _____.

This approach is in contrast with an approach providing the lexical item for number (I have *one* cat. I have *two* cats.) which makes the plural morpheme (*s*) redundant. Without the lexical indicator of number, the plural *s* is the only plural indicator in the above examples.

2. Teach possessive inflection of nouns in elliptical utterances, to place greater semantic load and stress on the inflection than it would receive within an utterance where word order + *Noun* (Mommy hat) signals possession.

   Clinician shows hat to child

   This hat belongs to Mommy.
   It is Mommy's hat.
   Whose hat is it?
   It is _____.

   Clinician points to big chair

   This chair is mine.
   Clinician points to small chair
   This chair is Jane's.
   Clinician points to appropriate chair as questions are asked
   Whose chair is this?
   It is _____.

3. Set up auxiliary and copular verbs (linking verbs) so that they carry maximum meaning by using variations in tense and number (the primary aspects of meaning carried by auxiliary and copular verbs).

   Clinician shows picture of one sheep

   Here *is* the sheep.

   Clinician shows picture of several sheep

   Here *are* the sheep.

   Clinician alternates pictures

   Show me the sheep. Here _____.
   Show me the sheep. Here _____.

   Capitalizing on meaning sometimes helps the child learn to include low-content words and keeps the clinician from admonishing "Don't forget to say *was*!"

4. Teach auxiliary verbs in utterance-final form to help furnish semantic clues and to yield maximum phonetic substance.

Clinician shows picture of boy running
The boy is running.
Clinician shows picture of boy sitting under a tree
The boy is not running now.
Is the boy running?
No, not now, but he *was.*
Is he running?
Not now, but he ____.

Many language-impaired children need to be shown how to modify previously adopted rules of linguistic structure that have prohibited their refinement of subclasses. Subclasses of morphemes, as well as other linguistic structures, mark subtle distinctions in meaning. In conversation, the speaker must indicate meaning differences, and the proper use of linguistic structures can help accomplish this task. Language-impaired children may need to be taught how to choose the most appropriate linguistic form to efficiently and accurately convey their meaning.

remediation of receptive deficiencies

Components of language are interdependent and as inseparable in intervention tasks as they are in normal acquisition. Separate discussions of language deficiencies in this book should not be taken to imply separateness among components or suggested sequence of intervention. "What to do" in intervention usually raises the problem of "what to work on first." There are at least two prevalent arguments regarding this problem:

> Developmental progression clearly advances from the level of understanding words to using words, reading words, and writing words (Myklebust, 1965; Wiig and Semel, 1976). The implication here is that intervention with language disorders should follow a developmental order in which remediation for language-processing deficits should precede remediation for language-production deficits (Berry, 1980; Wiig and Semel, 1980).

> Production and comprehension may proceed simultaneously in the development of normal children, or production may even lead comprehension in some areas (Vygotsky, 1962). This implies that intervention should include multilevel strategies and interactions among the various levels (Nelson, 1981).

Intervention with comprehension disorders does not necessarily have to precede, or exclude, intervention with expressive disorders (Nelson, 1981). In school-age children it is particularly difficult to isolate one aspect of language from another, and it seems undesirable to segment language except in discussion. Intervention with receptive deficiencies takes as many forms as permitted by the clinician's understanding of language, language deficits, and individual language disorders. Development of receptive language is one way in which the child organizes his/her world and experiences. A breakdown in receptive language can take many forms. The examples of intervention that follow illustrate the many directions intervention with language disorders can take.

Remediation of Receptive Disorders of Use Language impaired children with receptive disorders of use may have difficulty interpreting direct and indirect speech acts, participating in conversation as a responsive partner, and/or organizing their own behaviors and actions. The clinician must be creative in devising conversational situations in which the child can learn to interpret the verbal and nonverbal signals of the message and its intent, monitor the conversation to provide feedback to the speaker, and respond appropriately to the topic.

Interpreting Indirect Speech Acts

Help the child learn to interpret the intent of teasing comments or jokes.

> When Uncle Bob said, "I know Little Tommy doesn't want to go to the circus," he was teasing you. He said the opposite of what he knew you wanted to do, Tom, so he could make a joke with you. You could have said, "That's right. I *don't* like the circus," and made a joke back to him by saying the opposite of what you meant.

Help the child interpret indirect forms of request or instruction.

> Remember when I said, "Can you open the door?" I had my hands full of books, and I couldn't reach the doorknob. When I said that to you, I meant that I wanted you to open the door. I was asking if you would open it for me. People sometimes say things in such a way that the *words* have one meaning to you, but the *people* mean something else. You must look for what a person might mean other than what the words mean.
>
> John, when I said "I can't see the TV," I meant that the reason I couldn't see it was because you were in front of the TV. You stepped between me and the screen. I said that so you would move out of the way.
>
> Sometimes when people say, "Will you do something?" or "Can you do something?" they mean that they want you to do that and to do it then. If someone says "Do you think it's too cold?" they might mean that they want you to turn the air conditioner off because *they* are too cold.

Help the child learn contextual and nonverbal clues that influence the message or its intent.

Sue, when I frowned at you as I came into the room and said, "Is that any place to sit?" the frown and the question to you meant that I did not want you to sit on the table, and I wanted you to move. The frown meant I didn't like what you were doing, and the question told you what it was that I didn't like.

Matthew, when I winked at you and said, "I'll bet Jane doesn't want ice cream" that wink meant I was teasing. You and I were playing like Jane didn't want ice cream. Of course, we knew she did, because she had just clapped her hands when she saw the ice cream truck.

Participating as a Conversation Partner

Help the child use presuppositional clues to interpret utterances. World knowledge and contextual clues may be employed for interpretation.

When the TV advertisement says "You're a king when you drink Regals" it doesn't mean *you* are a king, because you're not. The name "Regal" means someone or something royal, like a queen or a king. The advertisement means that drinking a "Regal" soft drink makes you feel as important as if you were a queen or king.

Prior knowledge or shared speaker/listener knowledge may be used to interpret an utterance.

I just said, "*Our friend Bill* was here for class when you were out sick." You said, "Who's Bill?" Bill has been working with you in class for a long time. When someone uses a name, you must think whether they mean someone that you both know.

Help the child engage in dialogue through the use of feedback and revision strategies to repair communication breakdowns and through observance of turn-taking and topic maintenance.

1. *feedback and revision strategies* There are devices of dialogue for repairing communication breakdown that the child must learn to use and interpret. Often receptively-impaired children do not know they have misunderstood and do not give any clues about their misunderstanding. If it is apparent that the child has not understood the message or interpreted the intent correctly, he/she must be told that he/she did not "hear" all the words. ("The words were_____, and they meant_____.") The child should be instructed to say: "I didn't hear it" or "Say it again" when he/she does not receive the message clearly. It is important to teach the child how to respond to the entire message, and, when part of the message is obscured, to tell the speaker that clarification is needed. The child should be encouraged to say to the speaker:
   "Say it louder."
   "Say it again."
   "I didn't hear you."
   "I don't know what that means."

2. *turn-taking and topic maintenance* Often language-impaired children do not listen to their conversational partner's utterances, interrupting at will and speaking without consideration of the content or intent of the speaker's immediately preceding utterance. The clinician must help the child understand how to
a. Attend to the speaker: "Listen, Janet, she's still talking, and you can't talk while she is."
   "Wait Bill, don't ask me a question until I'm through telling you what to do."
b. Attend to the context: "Sallie, she asked you about the cut on your finger. Don't tell her about your new bike, until you've talked about your cut."

Intervention that addresses the reception of direct and indirect speech acts, participation in conversation, and repair of communication breakdown frequently requires metalinguistic skills.

"What did you *say?*"

"*Say* it again."

"*Tell* him to *say* it again."

"You can't *say* the same *thing* to Aunt Marilyn that you *say* to your brother."

"*Ask* me a *question.*"

"Did you hear *what I said?*"

The clinician needs to remember that metalinguistic skills themselves may need attention before (or as part of) the repair of conversational skills.

Remediation with Organizational Deficiencies

Children who cannot organize their behaviors and actions are probably demonstrating inadequate use of language for self-direction and control. They present a challenge to the intervention specialist and to their parents—whatever the source of the problem—because intervention requires that the child accept some responsibility for changing. Changing disorganized behavior and learning self-direction demands an extensive ongoing effort from children and their parents. Many attempts to help school-age children integrate their plans for carrying out tasks must involve compensation for the lack of automatic organizational skills. Work with parents and teachers must maintain this attention over time. If intervention is abandoned prematurely (at the first sign of improvement, for instance), or if anyone's efforts lag, then intervention loses its effectiveness.

Some of the approaches that seem to make a difference in children with organizational deficits include:

1. Organizing information from one channel (sensory pathway) to another
    a. *writing from dictation (numbers, letters, sounds, syllables, words, sentences)* Variations include length of utterance, timing of utterance as it is spoken, monitoring of correctness by self, clinician, and peers.
    b. *reading printed instructions and carrying out their directions* Variations include length, difficulty of instructions, instructions written correctly by clinician versus those written by another child with problems, speed of reading required.
    c. *carrying out spoken directions* Variations include length, difficulty of instructions, time span between hearing and acting, instructions given accurately by clinician versus those given by another child with problems, monitoring of actions by child or peers, type of response required (verbal, gross-motor, written).
2. Organizing life activities is
    a. *specifying and sequencing events that must be remembered and accomplished at home* Variations include keeping lists, charts, calendars, or schedules, which parents help monitor. Gradually the list becomes the responsibility of the child as the parents withdraw their reminders about it.
    b. *specifying and sequencing events that must be remembered and accomplished for school* Variations include recording study time, assignments given, assignments completed, assignments turned in, grades received, and teacher's notations on schedules or daily logs.
    c. *operating by clocks and timers* Variations include timing simple actions ("Set the timer for 15 minutes; when it goes off, come to the kitchen and show me that you have your socks and underwear on." "Set the timer for 15 more minutes, and, when it goes off, you must come to the kitchen table to eat.")

Any devices that focus the child's attention on the step-by step execution of a task and on the passage of time (whether or not the task is underway) should be beneficial in reducing the randomness of disorganized behavior. Consistent limits and predictable boundaries are important to children who cannot set their own limits or map their own actions. Older children sometimes can help each other in group therapy situations in which they describe problems in organization and action and attempt to resolve them.

Clinicians, parents and teachers may be able to help the disorganized child learn to compensate for lack of natural initiative and disorganization of life activities. Some older children and adolescents who have difficulty initiating or following through on tasks respond to structure for analyzing and monitoring their performance on various tasks. For example, they can learn to perform (1) task analysis, (2) time analysis and time structure, and (3) behavioral analysis and behavioral structure. Some ways of teaching children these analytical tasks include:

1. Task analysis
    a. Describe the end product.
    b. Describe the units and sequence of subtasks.

    c. Discuss ways of initiating the tasks (Tell the child that upon hearing the instruction to begin, he/she is to identify the first thing to be done.)

    d. Discuss ways of maintaining the task. (Use lists and schedules; describe ways of talking oneself through a task or action.)

    e. Discuss ways of monitoring tasks. (Teach the children to *observe* and *evaluate* each other's tasks and to be *initiators* for someone else, as in peer teaching.)

    f. Discuss ways of using strengths to shore up weaknesses. (Teach a non-visual learner or child with motor planning problems to talk himself/herself through a task: "First I get the right book; page 34, here it is. Then I put my name on the top of the paper real fast, and write down the problem numbers.")

2. Time analysis and time structure

    a. Discuss the amount of time needed for a task.

    b. Describe the use of time for self-competition. ("Can you do this assignment in ten minutes?")

    c. Give the children timers (or sandglasses) for their desks, and then limit their work time to specific duration, having them watch the passage of time as they work.

    d. Give the child less time than is needed for a task.

    e. Teach the child to analyze time/task units.

    f. Provide small groups with a timer designating a timekeeper for their group tasks.

    g. Let children discover how they need to use time. (Do they do better with no time constraints, or with rigid time limits?)

3. Behavioral analysis and behavioral structure

    a. Describe other people's actions, not in evaluative terms, but through observation and discussion.

    b Match impressions of other people's perceived actions. (Does Johnny describe Jim's actions more completely and accurately than Ben does?)

    c. Have the children learn to describe their own actions. (Tell how they looked, what they said, what movements they made, what reactions another person had to their behavior.)

    d. Discuss and act out social rules for behavior as demanded by the situation (school, parties), by audience (teachers, peers) and by conversational context.

It may benefit some children to hear specific rules of conduct or behavior, such as, "Do not touch someone else"; "Keep your voice soft"; "Ask someone else what *he'd* like to do"; "Keep appropriate distance and eye contact for the situation and listener."

One of the frustrating aspects of intervening with disorganized children is that unless the clinician or other monitoring person maintains contact with them the old disorganized behavior creeps back. It is important to keep the children in maintenance programs with external organization and structure until it is evident that they can monitor and modify their own actions on an ongoing basis.

Remediation of Receptive Disorders of Content Some school-age children do not refine their comprehension of classes of words and may fail to understand the distinctions in meaning that words convey. Comprehension deficits in school-age children may be difficult to remediate because they are hard to identify and describe. Echolalia has generally disappeared by the time children reach school age. Language-deficient children understand many utterances they hear, misleading the observer into thinking they understand "everything." Content-related intervention strategies with receptive disorders include the following:

1. Have the child demonstrate understanding of subclasses of words such as attributes (big-long, short-wide). Change the relationships among objects so that something once considered *big* is now considered *small*.
2. Create ways of helping the child organize his/her world into more discrete features through the understanding of word distinctions and tasks in word abstractions.
   a. What color is a blue bird?
   b. What kind of tree grows oranges?
   c. I'm holding a picture of a child. It's not a boy, so it must be a _____.
3. Teach the child to respond to low-content words that carry little information but clarify or specify elements of the message *(Give me the big, blue plane after you give me the little, red plane).*
4. Teach the child to listen to related utterances in a series rather than allowing responses based on the last thing spoken.
   a. Listen. My sister is at my house now. Later we'll go to the show. Where is my sister now?
   b. I had on my gloves and coat and boots. We were going to make a snowman outside. We stayed too long in the snow and got sick. Was it too cold or too hot outside?
   c. My brother was born three years before I was. He takes care of me when we go places, even though we're about the same size. Who is older, my brother or me?

Other content-related intervention strategies include:

1. Same-different judgments
2. Selection of a word from several choices
3. Sentence completion using appropriate word choice
4. Detection of absurdities in word use
5. Interpretation of ambiguous utterances from content

Remediation of Receptive Disorders of Form It seems that more programmed sequences of intervention and prepackaged kits have been produced for the phonological, morphological, and syntactical components of language than for any other component. For that reason, specific intervention ideas for reception of language form are not extensively covered in this book.

> Single components of language cannot be isolated for intervention, so that work on word order, for example, must also include relevant elements of meaning and their relations (for example, word sequencing in an utterance is not merely the proper combining of words, but involves the ways in which words relate to each other according to their meaning) (Miller and Yoder, 1972; Bloom and Lahey, 1978; Muma, 1978).

Specific items to work on for improvement of interpretation of form as it affects meaning for understanding include:

1. Variations of pronouns and verbs
2. Adjectives
3. Prepositions
4. Sentence type, length, and complexity
5. Meaning conveyed by the structural form

> For example, comprehension of morphemes is affected by the meaning the morpheme carries, the semantic role it signals, or the redundancies within the utterance that give the child more than one chance to understand its meaning. Morpheme meaning can be emphasized for the child by eliminating redundancy in the utterance, making the morphological change the only indicator of meaning.
>
> The clinician shows a picture of one cat and a picture of several cats, alternating the pictures and saying: We see the cat; we see the cats; show me the cat; show me the cats.

The same principle can be applied to other morphological markers in which the context forces the child to rely on the marker as the sole indicator of meaning.

> This hat belongs to Mommy.
> This is Mommy's hat.
> This is Mommy's.
> This is Daddy's hat.
> This is Daddy's.
> This is a picture of Mommy
> This is a picture of Daddy.

Show me the hat.

Show me Daddy.

Show me Mommy's hat.

Show me Daddy's.

disorders of written language

The following story is copied exactly as written by a thirteen-year-old boy with oral language deficiencies and a history of speech/language intervention and tutoring for academic subjects. In spite of at least average intellectual potential, the boy, and many others like him, continues to experience academic failure and frustration.

Oune long ago. Naoh sent out. Tew Aastrnots The Aastrnots mane was Jack, Bob they seaw somting the spice. This is thier stoy It started on 1960 Federary 20. Jack and Bob was blased in to space for two day was quite. The Dr Bell was testing thaer heet and bolood prise. One might Bob siad HELP! "Masion are heere Joe is out there mow fighting on with mastoin One is run blas us down Cap Goodnan sad bass them down

mext week the Clusin.

This stoy code be tre the mane was cangh to bite the incit

This story is true, and changing their names won't protect the innocent. But what is to be done about them?

There are many parallels between oral and written language. The categories of use, content, and form can be applied to both and frequently a deficiency in written language has a counterpart in oral language. A language-deficient child may read the words but not interpret the intent (use); misunderstand word meaning within the context (content); or fail to recognize a letter (form). Many of the comments made in previous sections regarding oral language can be applied to written language.

Theories regarding intervention with written language disorders are at least as varied as those dealing with oral language intervention. Specific programs have reported success at various levels. Some approaches to reading improvement emphasize the structure of the written word, including sound-letter association, grammatical and punctuation rules, word families, and sound blending. For example, Balow, Fuchs, and Kasban (1978) describe a remedial reading program in which each subject attended a basic-skill center every school day for 30 minutes over the course of 7 months. The skills approach involved the use of printed words that were analyzed for recurring visual patterns of letters. The authors found their program instructionally effective and attributed some of their program's successes to the fact that the children's attention was directed to the specific target (for example, word configuration).

Some current literature concentrates on the function of written language and urges that reading and writing be taught through a meaningful, useful approach. Jackson (1979), for example, delineates task-involvement situations in which the child acts out a story or actively participates in a situation. He/she must name words to describe the situation, put those words into written form in sentences, and read the sentences aloud. Miller (1976) describes a language-experience approach to reading intervention involving group-composed and individually dictated experience stories from which word charts are made. The children learn to understand reading as written talk.

Goodman (1976) writes that many remedial reading students are victims of "overskill." In describing reading comprehension, Goodman notes that since the purpose of language is communication, comprehension is integral to reading. Reading does not really exist without comprehension. One of Goodman's conclusions is that the use of phonetic analysis, to the exclusion of making sense of the sound combinations, can result in overemphasis on phonics and other word-attack skills in early reading instruction. Johnson (1976) also suggested that the emphasis in reading remediation should be on teaching children to look for meaning. This approach does not preclude the importance of phonics and word-attack skills, but does include emphasis on meaning in reading intervention.

Goodman (1976) and Johnson's (1976) position seems to be that efficient reading does not result from precise perception of all elements of the printed form but involves interaction between thought and language. Children begin speaking from a framework of meaning and not from a framework of sound analysis. Isolating language into fragmented skill units is a complex task for young speakers just as it is for young readers. It may be that the most natural learning sequence for reading begins with understanding the meaning of the sentence or phrase, progressing to comprehension of single words, and then sound-letter units. In oral language learning a speaker must differentiate the important from the unimportant. Some poor readers believe the only way to read a word is to be told the word by the teacher, or to sound out each letter as if it were just as important as the combination of letters. As Goodman (1976) notes, isolating sounds from words and words from connected phrases makes already-poor readers believe that each letter or word in reading is as significant as every other.

For example, many words are similar in configuration and young readers reverse the sequence of sound (reading *was* for *saw*). Many clinicians repeatedly make the child sound out the letter sequence with little long-term improvement of reading ability. However, if the child also learns to pay attention to the meaning of what is read, the intervention may be more effective.

Child (reading)	Clinician
We *was* a bird.	Does that make sense?
	What could that say that would make sense?
Oh . . . we *saw* a bird.	

Liberman, Shankweiler, Camp, Heifetz, and Werfelman (1977) report a developmental progression in the learning of auditory analytic skills. Children appear to progress from an ability to segment speech into words to an ability to segment words into sound, and finally, to an ability to segment syllables into sounds. Adequate speakers may not know that a word contains segments, because they hear the parts of spoken words almost simultaneously.

Explicit awareness and skills in segmentation as they apply to written form need to be taught to children. However, the danger in saying "sound it out" is that it may cause oversegmentation, distorting the word and masking its meaning in the utterance (Wallach and Stark, 1980). Sounding out the word "saw" (suh-aw-wuh), is an example of this type of distortion. Early reading parallels early speaking in many ways; intervention programs should heed these parallels. For example, predicting linguistic events in reading is as important as predicting linguistic events in speech. Readers must utilize their oral language knowledge of word meaning and word combinations, as well as phonetic analysis. Stories with meaningful, well-constructed sentences may be easier for a child to read than the simple, unpredictable baby-phrase combinations found in many primers. With well-constructed, predictable stories, the child can use information about possible word type, tense, and content in trying to predict approaching words.

One procedure designed to utilize semantic and syntactic aspects in the reading process is the cloze procedure described by Schlesinger (1968). A portion of the utterance is omitted, and the reader finishes the word, phrase, sentence, or story. Various adaptations of the cloze procedure have been used in both oral and written language intervention programs. For example, children are instructed to complete missing words in stories they have not read before, predict word endings, supply alternate words with similar meanings for a story they read, describe or change story endings, or determine complete words from partially spoken or printed words.

The variety of intervention approaches with written language disorders ranges from emphasis on sight reading to phonetic methods, to linguistic strategies in which word patterns and word families are stressed. Wiig and Semel (1980, pp. 376–386) provide an annotated summary of approaches to reading with specific reference to reading programs and reading materials. Some studies suggest that an increase in reading time alone will improve reading skills. Zigmond, Vallecorsa, and Leinhardt (1980) claim that very little school time is spent on activities contributing directly to growth in reading skills They suggest increasing reading time, particularly silent reading and discussion, for as little as five or ten minutes a day. They claim this small addition to reading time will significantly increase reading ability.

Language-impaired children transfer their oral language disabilities to the written form. If the child inadequately comprehends connected speech, he/she will inadequately comprehend written material. If the child does not draw conclusions well from conversation, then he/she will have difficulty with abstractions of written information. If the child cannot segment and analyze components of oral language well (sound segments, word differentiation and so on), then he/she will have the same problem with graphic representation of the language. Children with reading and writing problems need many of the same intervention strategies needed by children with oral language problems. They may require instruction in analyzing language components, refining subcategories of linguistic structures, deriving meaning from the entire context, determining if they have understood the material, and focusing their attention appropriately on the task.

Language intervention specialists should determine for themselves if intervention with written language disorders is to be included in their services. The specialist's decision may be influenced by his/her own knowledge of reading and writing tasks and ability to measure achievement and progress in reading, spelling, and writing, along with personal interest in written language disorders. Whether the language intervention specialist works directly with written language deficiencies or not, language is primary to reading, and written language disorders are legitimate territory for the language specialist.

selective attention

An important intervention task is directing language-deficient children in appropriate ways that focus their attention. Language-disordered children need to learn to direct their attention exclusively to the task or message, because it is unusual for a language-impaired child to be able to do two things at one time. If exclusive attention is not devoted to receiving the entire message (if for instance, the child is blowing his/her nose while the teacher is making an assignment), then the message may be missed. Evidently learning is facilitated when the child attends selectively. However, many language-impaired children find this an insurmountable obstacle without external monitoring ("Look at this"; "Listen"; "Pay attention"). Selective attention may be facilitated in the following ways:

1. Teaching the child to do one thing at a time (for example, to listen without moving, to organize a response before speaking, to be silent while carrying out an action).
2. Teach the child to rehearse internally what was heard until the message is clear or until it has been noted in another form (for instance, the pages in the math book have been marked).
3. Teach the child to begin something as soon as the information has been conveyed (for example, reject his/her request to "wait a minute" or "let me sharpen a pencil").
4. Limit the length of phrases and sentences in the instruction because the language-impaired child may have severe difficulty holding many thoughts in mind before beginning to lose some of the information (that is, give the child a short series of instructions and tasks and then check for completion, rather than giving him/her one long contract).
5. Use visual clues with verbal information.
6. Provide the language-impaired child with more than one repetition, task, instruction.
7. Remind parents and teachers to have the child "look" and "listen" before the message begins.
8. Counsel parents and teachers to eliminate background noises (talking, television, dishwasher, and so on) when the child is supposed to be listening.
9. Teach the child to picture the message in his/her mind as if he/she had a TV camera making pictures of the words heard or read.
10. Teach older children to monitor their own responses for accuracy (see section on using language to analyze language).

Clinician	*Child*
What did you just say?	I don't know.
What did I ask you to do?	To tell you what I did at school today.
Not quite. I said to tell me *two things* you did.	I wrote my words.
How many things did you tell me just now?	One thing.
Tell me another thing you did.	I ate my cheese sandwich.
Now how many things have you told me about what you did at school?	Two things.

○ INDIRECT INTERVENTION

Indirect intervention is a form of intervention in which the clinician advises others (parents, teachers, tutors) in the management of the language-impaired child. Parents, teachers, and peers are often discovered in disruptive or distorted interactions with language-deficient children. The cycle of noncommunication evolves in various ways.

1. In the presence of a speech, language, or hearing problem, the conveyance/ reception of the message between speaker and listener is often disrupted.
2. When the intended message is conveyed/received inadequately, the communication interchange is distorted.
3. Communication distortion or disruption interferes with interpersonal relationships and scholastic achievement.
4. The established difficulties in interpersonal and scholastic conditions contribute to additional communication distortions.

The Language of Interaction and Instruction Formal speech addressed to young children possesses many characteristics suggestive of tutoring. Adult speech to young children tends to be shorter, slower, and higher pitched than adult speech to older children (Bowerman, 1978). Parents and teachers of language-impaired children may need help in clarifying their messages to the children. Some parents and teachers do not notice that the children failed to understand what was said, nor do the parents modify their speech to the children. Young children and language-impaired children quit listening to utterances that are nonmeaningful to them. When children are pushed to the limits of their comprehension, they stop listening. Adults often do not realize that they have sprinkled their utterances with embedded clauses, innuendoes, metaphors, and other linguistically complicated forms. Some children grow up in environments with maids, very busy parents, or grandparents who have forgotten that children need to be taught various things. Normal language learners seem to learn language under any circumstances; language-deficient children may learn to talk in nonteaching environments, but may not learn the interpersonal functions of language.

Teachers often assume that children know and use a variety of vocabulary items, sentence constructions, concepts, and complex sequences of words. Teachers fail to recognize how difficult it is for language-impaired children to organize what they hear, and, therefore, how vital it is to repeat and reword instructions for such children (Wiig and Semel, 1980). For example, a child using short, simple sentence constructions has difficulty responding to math tasks requiring complex language structure. If a child does not understand the use of the word "and" as a connector of related words or utterances (although he/she may use the word "and" in spontaneous speech), he/she will have difficulty with the process of addition (Carlson, Gruenewald, and Nyberg, 1980).

Classroom language often affects the academic success of language-impaired children (Carlson et al., 1980). If a direction involves words with multiple meaning, is too long, or is given too rapidly, the language-deficient child may not catch its content. This can mean that additional details, given to enrich or illustrate the instruction, are more confusing than enlightening for the language-impaired child. The teacher may be able to adapt the language of classroom instruction for the language-deficient child without interfering with the teaching of other children. The language specialist may visit the classroom (or the resource room or the occupational therapist's room) to observe the teacher's instructional language so that he/she can suggest modifications. Visual aids, such as photographs and films, and aural aids, such as tape recorders for taping classroom lectures, may prove helpful to the teacher and the language-impaired child. Resource personnel might also help the teacher support the child, with oral tests and individual repetition of instructions to the child following the teacher's class presentations.

Schools have been careful to monitor the level of difficulty of subject matter, but little notice has been given to the complex nature of instruction the children receive. Language-impaired children may understand only parts of the instruction, or sometimes even tune out entirely the more complex messages (Berlin, Blank, Rose, and Rose, 1980). Although many classroom dialogues are designed to be preparatory to reading, the artificial compartmentalization of language into segments may interfere with a child's understanding of the way in which oral interaction actually develops. For example, in the classroom, the teacher may engage the class in a single-question/single-answer interaction, ignoring dialogue and feedback as ways of instruction.

If language-impaired children understand a lot of what is said to them, but miss subtleties of meaning or intentions, or if they do not recognize multiple meanings of words, they may need special consideration in situations where words are the primary means of communication (such as in the classroom). In classroom instruction and in other learning experiences, the speaker (teacher, mother, therapist) should know how to address the child in order to convey maximum information. The following suggestions may provide some guidance for those situations:

1. Use linguistic variations (say it a different way) when addressing children who do not understand everything they hear. Simple repetition or a louder voice may not help the child interpret the message. Changing the form of the utterance may help (for example, *Collect* the papers./ *Get all* the papers.)

2. Use nonverbal, demonstrable clues when possible to present information. Showing the child, gesturing, or acting out the message may help.

3. If the child is still echolalic, inhibit the echolalia by not allowing his/her repetition as an acceptable response. The child must demonstrate comprehension of the words you use by responding nonverbally (pointing, acting on the instruction, and so on).

4. Make all speech to the child concrete and direct. Avoid subtleties and innuendoes unless your specific task is to teach their meanings. Demonstrate the

new material, give examples, use visible and observable sign-to-symbol correspondences when possible, and set up situations in which the child must understand the message to succeed.

5. Never assume that the child understands the combined meanings of words in phrases and sentences, or that he/she understands words beyond his/her literal, referential meanings, even if he/she knows the meanings of the separate words you use. Change the tasks or situations to which the words apply so that you have opportunities to monitor the child's understanding of words in various contexts.

Parents and teachers sometimes become so confused by the interruptions in their interactions with the language-deficient child that even potentially successful activities do not occur. Some parents and teachers are unable to structure the simplest home or school situations for teaching the child things about language, the world, and conversation. Expectations about communication interactions, or biases about a person as a communication partner, can delay improvement in communication skills. People may begin to expect a child to speak, understand, and act in a deficient way and do not know how to help the child. Parents, teachers, and peers can participate in the intervention process in important ways.

1. Learn to understand the social and academic achievement difficulties imposed by language deficiencies.
2. Help the child and his/her family, teachers, and friends, to understand his/her strengths and minimize his/her obvious weaknesses.
3. Change the environment to facilitate learning and minimize barriers to increased communicative functioning.
4. Help the child take responsibility for changing and for compensating for deficiencies.

The purpose of this section is to illustrate ways to help parents, teachers, and language-impaired children themselves understand and manage the problems related to language deficiencies.

The clinician can help parents and teachers describe, understand, and focus on appropriate changes and expectations for the language-deficient child. He/she must not devalue parents' or teachers' efforts to help the child but he/she should provide information about and interpretation of the child's language behaviors. Parents must be able to understand the language disorder and its possible causes and perpetuating factors. Sometimes a better understanding of the deficiency allows them to deal with their own concerns about the child's language and/or behavioral inadequacies. If parents and teachers are instructed appropriately, they may learn to change the structure of their home or class and modify their interactions with the child. Parents and teachers also need help defining their own expectations for the child. Contact with the specialist who is intervening directly with the language deficiency is a golden opportunity for them to understand the problem and the intervention approaches, and to consider ways of mapping the child's academic and personal future.

understanding the problem

Questions from parents and teachers often demand that the clinician supply "answers." Parents have specific questions and want specific and definite answers; often the intervention specialist has few specific answers. One message the clinician should try to convey is that there are no definite solutions for cures. The questions parents and teachers ask reflect their frustrations. Clinicians can help them deal with the problems as they experience them. Questions to expect from parents and teachers include:

> What caused the problem?
>
> Should I change schools?
>
> What do you call the problem?
>
> Can you make her normal?
>
> I know he *can* do better than he does; why *doesn't* he?
>
> What can I do at home (at school) to help her?
>
> Why can't he do *anything* without constant supervision?

Discussing Language-Impaired Children with Teachers and Parents Teachers and parents frequently ask for a report describing the child's language-learning difficulties and how the language deficiency interferes with school and home life. Often the requests include questions regarding behavior, schoolwork, and discipline. Traditional means of reporting often do not meet the needs behind the request, and the clinician must find a useful way of reporting. He/she should use everyday words to explain learning deficiencies. The following examples may help clinicians develop their own everyday descriptions of language-learning disorders.

○ DESCRIBING LANGUAGE-LEARNING DEFICIENCIES TO PARENTS AND TEACHERS

1. *transmitting what he hears into what he does* John remembers what he hears quite well, unless he has to carry out the message physically. If he only has to repeat or understand what he hears, he does quite well; if he has to write or otherwise move as he hears the information, he is unable to retain it. This makes it difficult for him to write from dictation (spoken instruction he is expected to write down), or to move as the teacher gives directions ("Get out your math book, turn to page 44, and do the first line of problems").

2. *doing more than one thing at a time* If John is doing something with his hands or looking at something, he cannot attend to, or understand, what is being said to him. Teachers and family members must be sure that he is doing only one thing at a time if he is to understand and act appropriately.

3. *directing himself independently* John needs a lot of structure, routine, and consistency to help him map out and execute a plan of action. This includes planning how to do his homework, get his books home from school, show up at the right place at the right time, and play constructively and creatively. He is not a person who can organize automatically. Timing is not a "natural" skill, and organizing his life is difficult for him. He needs to learn to compensate for organizational problems with schedules, calendars, and checklists. His teachers must give him a series of short assignments instead of one long one He may need help in planning free time and in learning how to follow a schedule of appointments.

4. *analyzing what he sees* John has trouble looking at his own written work and determining if he has made any errors. This seems to reflect, in part, difficulty in moving his eyes together along a line of words. He skims a line, skipping letters and words without stopping to focus on each word and its accuracy.

Sometimes in describing a child's language-learning deficiencies and correlated academic problems, the vernacular of the profession's evaluation tools and philosophies interferes. Ways of describing disorders to school personnel who deal with the child include some of the following:

○ LANGUAGE-LEARNING DEFICIENCIES AND THEIR ACADEMIC CORRELATES

1. Some of Bill's academic problems seem to be related to his difficulty in making the transition from spoken to written language. Academic work requires that one learn to recognize the written counterpart of spoken sounds (sound-letter association in phonics, for example) and then represent spoken meaning in written form (reading and writing). If he only has to look at the letters and match them with other printed letters, he does well; if he only hears the sounds he can say the letter name. When he must transfer the sound "s" to the printed letter "s" his problems begin. Bill can blend sounds together to identify a word if no visual input is added. He cannot sound out printed letters and identify the word.

2. Other classroom behaviors illustrate Bill's difficulty integrating what he hears with what he does. For example, he has trouble if he is told to do something with his hands while the teacher describes what he is to do (Take your green pencils and draw two dots inside the yellow square).

3. It takes a lot of concentrated energy on Bill's part to keep his attention directed on what he should be doing. It is not easy for him to be on constant guard against distractions. Once disturbed by the slightest thing, he cannot continue

with a task, because he must concentrate fully to do anything with his hands. This means that a little scratch on his arm, another child's coughing, or the teacher's reminding the class to hurry, can bring his work to a complete stop. Without external guidance he cannot resume work.

Sometimes teachers have difficulty understanding the bases of language-learning deficiencies and doubt that a "real" problem exists. In many instances, however, teachers have less resistance to the learning interferences when they are described in terms of physical impairment (hearing or vision loss or other physical problems). When this is the circumstance, it may be more efficient for the clinician to discuss the language-learning disorder in ways that parallel sensory or physical deficits.

○ DESCRIBING LANGUAGE-LEARNING DEFICIENCIES AND ASSOCIATED PROBLEMS IN TERMS OF PHYSICAL IMPAIRMENT

1. Sallie has had problems since infancy with processing what she *hears*. She still has difficulty making sense out of words spoken in a group situation or when there is background *noise*. She *mis-hears* what is said to her and cannot listen well when she is doing anything other than totally concentrating on listening to and looking at the speaker. If she doesn't hear part of a word or sentence, she is not able to figure our what it might have been.

2. Sallie needs to be reminded to *watch* the teacher while instructions are being given. When she is working, she should be in the quietest part of the classroom. When possible, she should hear an *individual review* of the classwork and repeat her own understanding of new material and assignments.

Changing the Environment at Home *In some situations,* by the time intervention begins with school-age children, many parents are immobilized. They are overwhelmed and find it difficult to carry on ordinary parental teaching activities. They forget to stimulate the child with words for understanding and describing his/her experiences. They forget that they can play together with puzzles, activity books, and games, and can discuss movies. Parents often fail to use everyday situations like riding in a car or conversing at dinner to teach their children.

Parents must realize that tutoring and direct intervention work are not enough to help the child live with language-learning disabilities. They should be reminded sometimes of ways to make their home instructional, reinforcing, and predictable. The child will be more comfortable with a structure of firm rules and routines, without the tensions caused by loose structure and unexpected changes. The child must understand the terms for living within the family. He/she must learn that the terms are not negotiable to the extent of allowing him/her to get by without observing them and without participating in a productive way.

Many children with language-learning deficiencies need schedules and routines for everyday life and must become responsible for them. Frequently it is necessary to show them ways of compensating for disorganization through the use of charts, calendars, and checklists. Children often can carry out chores with the structure of a schedule requiring that each item be checked off as it is finished. They must usually be reminded to look at the list and check off the items, but this can be a step toward helping them be responsible for their duties.

Parents must discover ways to facilitate living with language-deficient children and to help the children learn at home. Some parents object to the suggestions regarding structure and firmness on the grounds that they do not want to be "mean" or "stifle" the child. Parents who object to setting consistent limits must be reminded that the child will be more comfortable and more functional only when the limits are predictable and the child not at the mercy of his/her disorganization. It is not kind to allow a child to live with inner chaos and expect him/her to act like everyone else.

Some of the following examples may help clinicians talk with parents about providing structure and consistency at home.

1. Have meals at the same time. Have chores, reading-time and bath-time in the same sequence.
2. Use a kitchen timer to help the child "see" time pass as he/she does routine activities like dressing and eating.
   "Watch the clock. When it gets here, we will clear the table and wash the plates. I hope you're through eating by then" (then be sure to do as you have said).
3. Prepare the child for changes.
   "Dad will be late tonight. We will watch T.V. first and then we will eat."
4. Limit his/her alternatives.
   "Here are two pair of pants. Which one do you want to wear today?"
5. Set up checklists.
   "Here is the checklist for your chores that we made together. Here is the checklist for your homework, with your class schedule by each day. Every night we'll look at them and see what you've checked off. Now, it's three o'clock. What can you begin doing now?"

Occasionally the checklists themselves become the obstacle to action because a child feels that item #2 cannot be started until item #1 is completed. Tell the child to do the items in order if possible, but to skip one if it cannot be done in sequence and return to that item later.

"Item #1 is feeding the cat. The cat is not here now, so you'll have to put that at the bottom of the list and go to item #2, which is picking up your underwear. You can do that now."

6. Help the child learn to prepare homework and classwork. For example, arrange to have the parents get the child's classwork assignments one day in advance so that the individual instruction done at home will be repeated in class. After an assignment has been accomplished in class, it should be reviewed at home and each assignment reread before the child begins homework.

Changing the Environment at School Classroom teachers rarely have time to devote extra effort to one child throughout the school year. It is stressful enough to have a language-impaired child in the classroom, to keep his/her attention, and to attempt to teach him/her the designated lessons while managing the rest of the class. However, many schools can supply part-time aids, resource teachers, or other special service personnel to help the teacher with the child and his/her special needs.

Since many language-impaired children require supervision and structure for optimal learning, teachers welcome suggestions for designing appropriate learning situations for the language-impaired children in the classroom. Some of the following examples should help teachers execute the necessary adaptations:

1. Beth seems to do best with support and supervision of her work. She is very poor at working independently and completing long-term assignments on her own. She works better with a short series of assignments than with long projects. She can complete one part at a time and show the teacher her understanding of the work, at which time the teacher can give Beth the next segment of the assignment.

2. Tim needs visual clues when he hears new information. These can include pictures, key words on the board, and/or visual examples of the information from the teacher. He understands the material if he experiences it rather than just hears about it (for example, if he went on a field trip to a fire station and discussed it, rather than merely hearing a story about a fire station). He needs to act out the meanings of words, see illustrations of theories, and so forth. Tim needs to learn to watch the teacher while he/she gives instruction or talks to the class. When he is working, he needs to be in the quietest part of the room. When possible, he must receive individual review of the classwork and his understanding of the assignments.

3. Jan must be reminded to "talk" herself through motor-planning and life-planning problems and to monitor her own organizational abilities. She needs to say to herself what she must do as if she were reviewing a sequence story. She must remember to picture in her mind what it is that must be performed and then match her actions to that visual image. She can learn to check her actions against the rehearsed actions to determine whether or not she accomplished the script she rehearsed.

Everyday Interactions at School

Many school-age language-deficient children cannot discuss, describe, or even identify their feelings and reactions. They may have simple sets of words such as angry or mad, happy or sleepy, but be unable to express more subtle distinctions. When they become anxious, frustrated, or physically uncomfortable they often become irritable, weepy, or physically aggressive. Classroom teachers can help language-deficient children identify and express their reactions by finding opportunities to talk about their feelings and supplying the words for discussing them. This can occur without interferring with the behavior limits that need to be reinforced.

1. I know you're angry with me. I get angry, too. I still like you, and after you're not feeling so angry about your grade, we'll talk about it.

2. You're surprised and angry because you didn't expect Bobby to run up and grab you and hug you. You don't like surprise hugs, and it doesn't feel good. But Bobby doesn't know that. He likes you and wanted to show you he does; he didn't know he would hurt your arm.

3. You're worried about the testing and feeling a little afraid that you cannot make good grades. You said you're dumb, but I know you're not; in fact, you are very smart in most things. In a very few ways you have trouble remembering things, like spelling words, but that doesn't mean you're dumb.

Children need to try to verbalize their feelings instead of engaging in violent reaction or complete withdrawal as their only alternative responses. Sometimes it is difficult for teachers and parents to acknowledge children's feelings when their behavior is unacceptable. It is necessary, however, to help children learn words for expressing their feelings and learn appropriate ways of acting on those feelings.

It is difficult to encapsulate important suggestions for home and school management of the language-deficient child. As soon as we identify specific ways of helping some children, we find that those ways do not work with other children. Living with and teaching language-impaired children and adolescents involves complex dynamics that often are unpredictable. Some sample suggestions for clinicians to consider when discussing the management of language-deficient children with parents and teachers are listed below.

sample suggestions for management of language-impaired children at school

1. Structure, routine, and consistency are vital to language-deficient children. External means of preparation and organization are necessary, such as calendars, lists, and schedules. Surprises and unstructured situations are overstimulating and leave many children with extra, undirected energy.

2. Repeat all instructions to the class. After the class has received the instructions or assignment, give the instructions to the child individually.

3. Repeat instructions if a noise occurs while instructing the class (a book falls, a child coughs, and so forth). Do not give assignments while there is outside noise (children in the hall), because the child might have trouble filtering background noise from the sound of teacher's voice.

4. Give the child short assignments in a series, rather than one long one. Recheck the child's understanding of the material at the end of each segment of work and provide reinstruction as necessary.

5. Remember that *talking with* language-impaired children is not equivalent to *communicating.* Because a child hears and a teacher talks, does not mean that the child understands and can carry out the instruction.

6. Visual and experiential demonstrations must be provided when possible, because language-deficient children will not learn optimally from information that they have only heard.

7. Do not let the language-deficient child do anything while giving him/her instructions. Frequently language-deficient children cannot attend to what they hear if they are doing anything else.

8. Allow the child to work alone and not in groups. Take care that the separation of the child from group work does not look like punishment, but merely a convenience for him/her. The child will benefit from one other child or an aid helping to monitor the progress of independent work.

9. The language-deficient child must have a place in a notebook (a calendar with daily subject and time blocks) to record each assignment in each class and to check off the completion of that assignment.

10. Permit the child to take tests orally if you are concerned about the child's level of information, and he/she cannot perform well on written examinations.

11. Do not allow the child's mimicry of new material to serve as the only indicator of what he/she understands about the information. Have him/her rephrase the information or otherwise demonstrate understanding of new material.

sample suggestions for management of language-impaired children at home

1. Structure, routine, and consistency are usually beneficial for children with language-learning problems. Try to keep as much sameness for your child as possible. This includes having meals about the same time in the same way every day, having daily schedules in predictable order, and following routines for dressing, eating, and bathing.

2. If an unpleasant job or time-consuming task must be undertaken, set a timer for the child to watch. Providing time markers to make the passage of time seem more related to the production of a task can help a child focus on a task and can give him/her a way of initiating activity. (For instance, set a timer for 10 minutes, and show the child that when it gets "here" it will ring, and the child is to come to the kitchen with blouse and shorts on.)

3. Try to avoid surprises for the young language-impaired child. Unexpected, noisy, or busy situations, such as surprise parties, trips, unannounced company, or unexpected absences can be very upsetting. If the child becomes overly aggressive in stimulating circumstances, remove him/her from the busy situation, calm him/her, and redirect his/her attention.

4. Some children with language disorders have related problems, including difficulty interpreting touch or movement. Your child may not like physical contact unless he/she initiates it and may find many physical sensations (types of clothes, showers, hair brushing, tickling and so on) very uncomfortable.

5. Try to emphasize strengths and minimize weaknesses. Instead of saying, "You can't do that. You make a mess of it every time." say "You do *this* so well; I need your help here instead."

6. Be sure your child does not overhear your discussions about him/her. You can talk with him/her directly about their good points, and explain simply the behaviors that work.

7. Your child may not be able to concentrate with background noise or other distractions. If you have something to say, turn down the TV and ask the child to look at you.

8. Your child may need your reassurances about his/her abilities. Many children have fantasies about themselves that are more frightening than anything they could be told about their learning impairment.

9. If your child has difficulty remembering what he/she hears, try to keep your instructions to him/her as short as possible. Tell him to picture each part of an instruction as if he/she had a TV camera in his brain taking pictures of what he/she hears.

10. When possible, provide his/her own room or at least a place that belongs to him/her. Teach him/her to retreat to the room when things become "too much."

11. The child may have tantrums and overreact to minor problems. Many things contribute to inappropriate emotional outbursts. Parents should work with the clinician regarding specific problems.

12. Do not allow the child to make open-ended decisions; provide choices for him/her. The child will be happier and respond more quickly if you give him/her ways to make decisions. (Do you want to wear the green shirt or the red one? Do you want to buy the chocolate ice cream or the strawberry? Do not say: What do you want to wear? Which ice cream do you want?)

13. Help the child adjust to new situations by talking about an approaching change before it occurs. (in dinner plans, school schedules, company, and so on). Getting into and out of routines, such as on holidays, may make the child's behavior and general functioning appear to deteriorate.

14. Help the child break down large tasks (Clean your room.) into small, manageable segments. (Pick up your socks; now, put your dirty clothes in the clothes hamper; now, put all your books on the desk.)

referrals and resources

Language-impaired children and adolescents frequently present problems requiring more services than any single profession can provide. Intervention programs should include well-coordinated patient care from many professions. It is unusual to find a language-deficient child who requires only the services of a language specialist. Frequently professionals with other expertise are needed.

Every clinician should have a resource list of available community services that language-deficient people might require. These may include medical specialists, teachers and tutors with special expertise with language-deficient children, private and public schools that offer particular structures or programs, vocational and trade schools; and other professional specialists. The list will be valuable for making efficient and appropriate referrals and for seeking advice from persons with various skills regarding a particular child's needs. Two of the most important nonmedical professionals in my intervention with language-deficient children have been the psychologist and the sensory integration specialist.

The Psychologist A psychologist who understands normal child development as differentiated from abnormal child development, who has a working knowledge of language-learning deficiencies, and who is sensitive to the communication processes of human interaction can offer valuable help in at least the following ways:

1. *Assessment* In working with language-learning-deficient children, it is sometimes difficult to determine which components of human behavior are interfering with normal communication. The psychologist can assist with:
   a. Intellectual assessment to help decide whether the child has a specific deficiency in certain aspects of learning, with strength in nonimpaired areas, or if the child is globally slow or retarded
   b. psychodiagnostic evaluation to determine whether the child's interactions and responses are appropriate within the world as perceived through learning deficiencies, or if the child's interpersonal distortions are based on some type of specific emotional disturbance

Jack's mother brought him for speech/language evaluation when he was three years old, reporting that his speech was generally accurate in inflection, grammar, and pronunciation. She was concerned that Jack often did not make sense when he spoke and seemed unaware that what he said was nonsensical. When Jack behaved inappropriately, acting as his mother termed, "bizarre" (having a totally different conversation from his listener), she worried that Jack was disturbed and out of contact with reality.

The speech/language pathologist referred the child to a psychotherapist for psychodiagnostic assessment. The psychologist's evaluation and observations led her to the conclusion that Jack was not psychotic, and was operating as appropriately as he could within the framework of the language deficiencies.

An intensive language intervention program based on semantic and pragmatic components of communication was begun. Two years later, Jack was doing well in kindergarten, making friends, and behaving appropriately for his age.

2. *Patient Counseling and Psychotherapy* Often the language-impaired child exhibits behavioral and emotional disruptions in addition to language-learning deficiencies. The psychotherapist (used here to describe a psychologist with training in clinical psychology and psychotherapy) can work with the language remediation specialist in helping the child through various adjustment difficulties and in guiding the child's family through the disruptions and chaos of family life with an impaired child.

The psychologist can help older language-deficient children accept responsibility for coping with their problems and making changes that will help them deal with their deficiencies. We recognize the truth and frustration in a child who screams "You don't understand me!" None of us really understands what it is like to live with severe language-learning deficiencies. This very fact makes it important for language-deficient children to learn that they must do a lot of the changing themselves. The child must accept ultimate responsibility for personal actions. The world is not going to change to excuse deficiencies nor allow for extra efforts needed to function in certain situations. The psychotherapist gives the child the support and the opportunity for reality testing needed for these painful acknowledgements.

3. *Parent and Family Support and Counseling* The stresses a language-deficient child creates for parents and the family unit vary with the nature of the language disorder and the child, but stress is a reality. The family experiences stress in having to relinquish some of their time together, because the child makes that time miserable for everyone; in having to provide extra help and time with homework; in experiencing public embarrassment over the child's behavior; and in worrying about the child's academic failure. At every stage of development, the child with severe language-learning deficiencies needs parents who are firm, who specify and enforce the rules of living together, and who are able to avoid the marital conflicts a language-impaired child can exacerbate. The constancy of the child's demands may seem intolerable at times.

Symptoms of the language-learning deficiency change with age, but the stresses remain. When the child is young, he/she may sleep in the parents' bed because of night fears or because of his/her need for physical support; parents may not get the child into his/her own bed for several years. As the child grows older, he/she may have difficulty making friends in school, experience problems with academic achievement, fail to bring homework home or turn in assignments, and eventually be unable to keep a job.

The psychotherapist can help parents recognize some of their own personal and marital conflicts, which are heightened by the language-deficient child; deal with their own grief and conflict regarding their child; and learn to structure their lives to provide a home environment beneficial for the child and tolerable for themselves.

The Sensory Integration Specialist Some of the earliest concerns parents voice about their children are related to physical well-being and behavior. Beyond guarding their child's immediate health, they may not know what kind of treatment, observation, or assistance is most effective. They may not understand symptoms or the implications of deviations in motor development or coordination.

Occupational therapists or physical therapists specializing in sensory integration (Ayres, 1976; 1980) or developmental disabilities can help

diagnose and intervene with visual-motor and motor-development inadequacies. These specialists may assist in analyzing motor problems from early
infancy through childhood and adolescence, and, in certain instances,
throughout adult life. They may identify problems of processing and integrating information received from touch, from body position and movement, and from the way the child interprets what is seen or felt. They may
recognize a child's inadequacies in the way the body plans and carries out
movement through small and large motor actions.

Early complaints about these problems may be described as an infant's
irritability at being moved, held, or touched; poor development of motor
skills; and/or late acquisition of motor milestones. Some parents report
that their children dislike being hugged unless they initiate the physical
contact. They say that these children cannot tolerate touching anything
fuzzy, won't wear certain clothes, won't go barefoot in the grass, and will
fight against having their hair washed. Trips to the barber may be hor-
rible experiences for the child and family because of the child's objection
to being touched. It is interesting to note that children who cannot tolerate
and interpret certain touch or movement experiences seem to need extra
touch and movement of their own choosing. They turn in circles for very
long periods of time, rub their skin raw, or rock and bang their heads. They
seem to require stronger physical input than most children do, but respond
with primitive defensive behavior if the input is out of their control (for
example, if someone approaches them to hug them, they may recoil or
wince).

Children with tactile problems often act as if they are not affectionate, and
their parents often feel rebuffed when their child refuses their expressions
of affection. Parents need to know that the child can come to them with
physical affection on his/her own terms for touching, but that he/she may
not be able to tolerate their initiation of physical contact. They should
understand that a child with tactile problems (sometimes called "tactilly
defensive," Ayres, 1976) does not seem to accurately interpret the sensation
of being touched and reacts to unexpected or unseen touch as if it were very
uncomfortable.

As certain language-deficient children get older, their physical activity
seems disorganized, and their general motor behavior appears undirected.
They may be excessively active and unable to do any one thing for more than
a few minutes at a time. Some children look clumsy or act as if they are not
put together very well physically. Some of these children cannot eat a meal
or put on their clothes without constant supervision, appearing incapable
of executing a series of simple motor acts. Some children are disoriented
by sudden movements such as an unexpected turn, a jostle from someone,
or a fall. These children may be disoriented in new environments, fall from
chairs unexpectedly, and panic at swimming pools or on carnival rides.
Certain visual-motor problems may make it very difficult to participate in

certain sports. For example, soccer may be a good choice for a child with poor eye-hand coordination because that child may have good eye-foot coordination. Baseball, on the other hand, can be a very bad experience for a child with poor eye-hand coordination.

The occupational or physical therapist trained in testing and observing developmental motor functioning can assess a child's adequacies in tactile/visual-motor/motor behaviors:

Assessment The sensory integration specialist can describe problems in visual-motor skills, gross and fine motor performance, and tactile-proprioceptive functioning (skin and muscle feedback from external input). Occupational therapists are employed at my own speech/language center because of the high incidence of motor control or motor planning problems in our population of communicatively impaired children. They intervene with the motor integration problems of infants, preschool and school-age children, and young adults. Through their assessment of infants with motor disabilities, they also help identify those who may be a high risk for other problems (for example, language-learning disorders).

Intervention Sensory integration programs usually are based on evaluation of the body's organization of the world and are designed to help children organize their movements, react appropriately to movement and visual input, and understand the relationship between their bodies and the physical world. Therapeutic goals may include improving gross and fine motor coordination, planning and executing a series of physical movements, and improving the child's general physical adaptation to the environment.

Parent Information and Direction Frequently a sensory integration specialist can assist the language remediation specialist, parents, and teachers regarding the child's behaviors as they relate to developmental motor coordination and tactile problems. For example, a child who is defensive about being touched may: (a) wiggle constantly when seated; (b) look continuously to see what may be nearby that could touch him/her; or, (c) react aggressively if a child accidentally or playfully bumps him.

Parents and teachers need to recognize behaviors that are characteristic of children who do not know how to interpret their physical world. They also need suggestions about how to make children more comfortable physically. For example, children with tactile defensiveness seem to become very uncomfortable when they must sit in chairs for very long. They act, after five minutes in a wooden chair, like they've been six hours on a bed of needles. Their tolerance for sustained physical pressure seems very minimal and interferes with attention to any other input, such as the teacher's instruction. Children with problems interpreting touch often display enormous reactions to minor accidents, such as crying with anger or agony at the slightest scratch.

There are some ways of making a child with these problems more comfortable and more receptive to input. This involves redirecting his/her attention away from what might touch him/her to the input itself, by providing him/her with such aids as the following:

> Place a cushion on the child's chair for him/her to sit on to relieve the pressure of the chair against his/her legs. The discomfort of hard chairs and the requirement of staying in one place can be intolerable for tactilly defensive children.
>
> Seat the child in the front quarter of the classroom, near a side wall so his/her chair can be angled toward the teacher. This arrangement places the child in a position from which he/she can see the teacher and most of the class in one visual field. Many overactive children are mistakenly placed next to the teacher's desk with their backs to the class so the teacher can keep the child's attention and avoid distractions for him/her. The effect of this arrangement is that the child feels compelled to turn toward the class constantly to check out every sound.

Some parents and teachers feel that self-discipline and willpower are the most deficient qualities in unmanageable children. Undoubtedly there is some truth to this, however, language-impaired children with related problems of motor or tactile disorders need some external aid to their will power. It may be necessary to phrase descriptions of the child's problems in terms of their physical correlates to engage teachers' help.

> Sam has had some joint and muscle problems and often is physically uncomfortable. His tendency to move in his chair, sit on his knees, and stand up are attempts to make his body more comfortable. When he is uncomfortable, he becomes excessively active and does not attend properly to classroom work. He needs to have a cushion on his chair and to have a chair from which his feet can touch the floor. When he asks to sharpen his pencil or to get a drink, that means he feels he needs to move a little. He should be allowed to do so. If he chooses to stand at his desk to do his work, he needs to be permitted to do this. His desk should be placed near a wall so that he can see the teacher and the rest of the class without worrying that someone will bump into him.
>
> Jane's vision interferes with her work because her eyes cannot follow a line smoothly across a page, and she cannot shift well from looking at the board to looking at her own paper. If the glare on the board is such that she cannot see part of the letter or word, she is unable to visualize what the entire letter or word is. She needs help in checking her copying work in case her eyes have played tricks on her.

The sensory integration specialist can help clinicians, parents, and teachers understand sensory-motor integration and visual-motor dysfunction and their influence on a child's learning patterns and behaviors. This specialist can intervene, prognosticate future functioning, and assist with aspects of learning problems based on visual-motor perception, touch, and movement. These influences on the child should be considered when establishing educational and social goals.

The Tutor   Academic skills and academic failures of language learning-deficient children frequently are the target of concern. Sometimes we must make decisions regarding the referral of a child for tutoring. Both tutoring and therapy are forms of intervention and are not mutually exclusive. However, when poor grades become the chief complaint about school-age children, the intervention program may need to incorporate direct tutoring with academic material. The language specialist may be qualified to tutor the child on academic subjects as part of the language intervention program, or a tutor may be needed.

Tutorial intervention is usually directed at academic skills needed to accomplish specific subject-related goals (for instance, the multiplication tables, third-grade reading). The instruction itself can be individualized and structured, directing the child's attention to the material through repetition and re-instruction. Tutoring often implies the teaching of splinter skills— teaching a task with little regard to the underlying basis of competence (sight reading, articulation drill, penmanship, and so forth). Some tutoring programs coordinate the task drills with attempts to alleviate the disruption in learning processes that apparently interferes with achievement. Tutoring of this nature seems more therapeutic because of the generalizations about "how to learn" that may transfer to other subject matter. Effective tutoring can be a beneficial aspect of intervention; poor tutoring can be a regrettable substitute for more basic intervention.

○ THE PROCESS OF INTERVENTION

The core of direct intervention lies in the way the clinician deals with what the children bring to the situation. The clinician has to seize every teaching opportunity, by using the child's readiness and responses, by employing what the child brings to the session both linguistically and personally, and by adapting readiness and reaction to the intervention goals. In order for this process to occur, the intervention specialist must be an expert in the use of language and in analyzing the language skills of others.

the clinician in the intervention process

The clinician must apply his/her own knowledge of communication in the intervention process to change those very features in which the child is deficient. If the clinician is deficient in any component of language, then he/she should not engage in direct language intervention.

Some student clinicians become proficient in language analysis, but their own style of language in communicative interactions interferes with their effectiveness. A clinician's interpersonal skills affect the dynamics of the intervention process, but often it is difficult to document and change an adult's interpersonal behaviors. Supervisors of training programs frequently have trouble justifying their objections to some of the students-in-training whose academic proficiencies are impeccable but whose poor interactive skills interfere with the sensitive dynamics of therapeutic situations. Equally difficult to justify are the students who do not achieve high scores in academic areas but who have an innate excellence in clinical work.

It seems reasonable to assume that if a clinician is to assess and remediate disorders of language use, content, and form, he/she should possess those communicative skills. Practicing clinicians and students-in-training might subject themselves to the same analyses they apply to language-deficient children.

1. Does the clinician *understand* the process of intervention in terms of prioritizing and changing aspects of the intervention program?
2. Will the clinician *organize* the intervention format in terms of long- and short-term planning, adapting to the child's changes?
3. Does the clinician apply appropriate intervention *structure* to the child's needs at each stage of intervention through direct and indirect intervention and proper use of resources and referrals?
4. Does the clinician apply appropriate *content* in the intervention program based on knowledge of language and language deficiencies?
5. Does the clinician apply appropriate *use* of communication behaviors in clinical interactions with the child, for analysis of the child's language, and for interaction with the child's parents and teachers?

Differences in intervention strategies and style vary with differences in clinicians; the most effective clinicians develop their own styles, learning from their teachers and peers without emulating another clinician's words or movements. Great clinicians often are lauded for their teaching techniques or methods. It is probable, however, that great clinicians would be great regardless of the content or methods they adopted because of the professional-and-person-specific features they use in the process of intervention.

Intervention represents a highly developed level of communicative interaction; there is no prefabricated routine to follow with any child, no safety in experience, and no room for a technician. Simple problems and simple solutions are rare. Successful intervention with language-impaired children and adolescents requires a linguistically competent person, as well as a professionally competent clinician, who accepts long-term responsibility for each person with whom intervention is attempted.

SUMMARY

Language deficiencies and related disorders are not always eliminated in people who have participated in intervention programs. Some studies indicate that even after intervention, some language-impaired children and adolescents have difficulty with school achievement and social interactions (Hall and Tomblin, 1978; Sheridan and Peckham, 1978; Weiner, 1974). However, recent reports suggest that current intervention strategies result in marked improvement in language-impaired children who receive early intervention (Snyder, 1980). The suggestion to "wait and see" and comments such as "He'll outgrow it by ten or twelve" are not always based on sound judgment about communicative competence or knowledge of current intervention processes. Any parent or teacher who continues to be concerned about a child's language development or school achievement should pursue help for the child until satisfied that appropriate identification and intervention have been provided. Intervention can facilitate more adequate language behaviors and minimize deficiencies in language-impaired people.

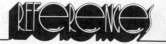

ALLEN, D., L. BLISS, and J. TIMMONS, "Language Evaluation: Science or Art?," *Journal of Speech and Hearing Disorders,* 46 (1981), 66–68.

AMERICAN SPEECH AND HEARING ASSOCIATION COMMITTEE ON LANGUAGE, "Meeting the Needs of Children and Adults with Disorders of Language: The Role of the Speech Pathologist and Audiologist," *Asha,* 17, (1975), 273–78.

AMERICAN SPEECH AND HEARING ASSOCIATION COMMITTEE ON LANGUAGE LEARNING DISABILITIES, "The Role of the Speech-Language Pathologist in Learning Disabilities," *Asha,* 22, (August 1980), 628–36.

ARAM, D. and J. NATION, "Patterns of Language Behavior in Children with Developmental Language Disorders," *Journal of Speech and Hearing Research,* 18, (1975), 229–41.

AUSTIN, J., *How to Do Things with Words.* Cambridge, Mass.: Harvard University Press, 1962.

AYRES, J., *Sensory Integration and Learning Disorders.* New York: Academic Press, 1976.

AYRES, J., *Sensory Integration and the Child.* Los Angeles: Western Psychological Services, 1980.

BAKER, H. and B. LELAND, *Detroit Tests of Learning Aptitude.* Indianapolis: Bobbs-Merrill, 1967.

BALOW, B., D. FUCHS, and M. KASBAN, "Teaching Non-readers to Read: An Evaluation of the Basic Skills Centers in Minneapolis," *Journal of Learning Disabilities,* 11, no. 6 (June–July 1978), 351–54.

BANGS, T., *Language and Learning Disorders of the Pre-Academic Child: With Curriculum Guide.* New York: Appleton-Century-Crofts, 1968.

BANGS, T., *Language and Learning Disorders of the Pre-Academic Child: With Curriculum Guide.* 2nd Edition. Prentice-Hall, 1982.

BATES, E., "Pragmatics and Socio-linguistics in Child Language," in *Normal and Deficient Child Language,* edited by D. Morehead and A. Morehead. Baltimore: University Park Press, 1976, pp. 411–63.

BEILIN, M., *Studies in the Cognitive Basis of Language Development.* New York: Academic Press, 1975.

BENDER, L., *Bender Motor Gestalt Test.* American Orthopsychiatric Association, 1946.

BENTON, A. and D. PEARL, eds., *Dyslexia: An Appraisal of Current Knowledge.* New York: Oxford University Press, 1978.

BERKO GLEASON, J. and S. WEINTRAUB, "Input Language and Acquisition of Communicative Competence," in *Children's Language,* vol. 1. Edited by K. Nelson. New York: Gardner Press, 1978.

BERLIN, L., M. BLANK, M. ROSE, and S. ROSE, "The Language of Instruction: The

Hidden Complexities," *Topics in Language Disorders*, 1, no. 1 (December 1980), 47–58. Edited by K. Butler and G. Wallach. Rockville, Md.: Aspen Systems.

BERNSTEIN, B., *Class, Codes and Control:* vol. I. Theoretical Studies Toward A Sociology of Language. London: Routledge and Kegan Paul, 1972.

BERRY, M., *Language Disorders of Children: Bases and Diagnoses.* New York: Appleton-Century-Crofts, 1969.

BERRY, M., *Teaching Linguistically Handicapped Children.* Englewood Cliffs, N.J.: Prentice-Hall, 1980.

BLACHOWICZ, C., "Semantic Constructivity in Children's Comprehension," *Reading Research Quarterly*, 13, (1977–78), 187–99.

BLANK, N., Review of *Toward an Understanding of Dyslexia*, by F. Vellutino in *Dyslexia: An Appraisal of Current Knowledge*, edited by A. Benton and D. Pearl. New York: Oxford University Press, 1978, pp. 115–17.

BLANK, N. and E. FRANKLIN, "Dialogue with Preschoolers: A Cognitively-Based System of Assessment," *Applied Psycholinguistics*, 1, no. 2 (1980), 127–50.

BLOOM, L., *Language Development: Form and Function in Emerging Grammars.* Cambridge, Mass.: MIT Press, 1970.

BLOOM, L., "Talking, Understanding and Thinking," in *Language Perspectives: Acquisition, Retardation and Intervention*, edited by R. Schiefelbusch and L. Lloyd. Baltimore: University Park Press, 1974, pp. 285–312.

BLOOM, L., *Readings in Language Development.* New York: Wiley, 1978.

BLOOM, L. and M. LAHEY, *Language Development and Language Disorders.* New York: Wiley, 1978.

BOEHM, A., *The Boehm Test of Basic Concepts.* New York: Psychology Corporation, 1970.

BOWERMAN, M., "Semantic Factors in the Acquisition of Rules for Word Use and Sentence Construction," in *Normal and Deficient Child Language*, edited by D. Morehead and A. Morehead. Baltimore: University Park Press, 1976, pp. 99–179.

BOWERMAN, M., "Semantic and Syntactic Development: A Review of What, When and How in Language Acquisition," in *Bases of Language Intervention*, edited by R. Schiefelbusch. Baltimore: University Park Press, 1978, pp. 97–190.

BRANSFORD, J. and K. NITSCH, "Coming to Understand Things We Could Not Previously Understand," in *Speech and Language in the Laboratory, School, and the Clinic*, edited by J. Kavanagh and W. Strange. Cambridge, Mass.: MIT Press, 1978, pp. 167–307.

BROWN, R., "The First Sentences of Child and Chimpanzee," in *Psycholinguistics*, edited by R. Brown. New York: The Free Press, 1970.

BROWN, R., *A First Language: The Early Stages.* Cambridge, Mass.: Harvard University Press, 1973.

BRYAN, T., "Social Relationships and Verbal Interactions of Learning Disabled Children," *Journal of Learning Disabilities*, 7, (1978), 107–15.

BRYAN, T. and F. PFLAUM, "Linguistic, Cognitive and Social Analyses of Learning

Disabled Children's Interactions," *Learning Disability Quarterly,* 1, (1978), 70–79.

BURROWS, T. and D. NEYLAND, "Reading Skills, Auditory Comprehension of Language, and Academic Achievement," *Journal of Speech and Hearing Disorders,* 4, (November 1978), 167–472.

CALFEE, R., R. CHAPMAN, and R. VENEZKY, "How a Child Needs to Think to Learn to Read," in *Cognition in Learning and Memory,* edited by L. Gregg. New York: Wiley, 1972, pp. 139–82.

CARLSON, J., L. GRUENWALD, and B. NYBERG, "Everyday Math is a Story Problem: The Language of the Curriculum," *Topics in Language Disorders,* 1, no. 1 (December 1980), 59–70. Edited by K. Butler and G. Wallach, Rockville, Md.: Aspen Systems.

CARROLL, J., "Developmental Parameters of Reading Comprehension," in *Cognition, Curriculum and Comprehension,* edited by J. Guthrie. Newark, Del.: International Reading Association, 1977, pp. 1-15.

CARROLL, J., "Thought and Language," in *Thought and Language/Language and Reading,* edited by M. Wolf, M. McQuillan and E. Radwin. Cambridge, Mass.: Harvard Educational Review, 1980, pp. 626–31.

CARROW, E., *Test of Auditory Comprehension of Language.* Austin, Texas: Learning Concepts, 1973.

CARROW, E., *Carrow Elicited Language Inventory.* Austin, Texas: Learning Concepts, 1974.

CAZDEN, C., *Child Language in Education.* New York: Holt, Rinehart, and Winston, 1972.

CHAFE, W., *Meaning and the Structure of Language.* Chicago: University of Chicago Press, 1970.

CHAPMAN, R., "Comprehension Strategies in Children," in *Speech and Language in the Laboratory, School, and Clinic,* edited by J. Kavanagh and W. Strange. Cambridge, Mass.: MIT Press, 1978, pp. 308–27.

CHOMSKY, C., *The Acquisition of Syntax in Children from Five to Ten.* Cambridge, Mass.: MIT Press, 1969.

CLARK, E., "What's in a Word? On the Child's Acquisition of Semantics in His First Language," in *Cognitive Development and the Acquisition of Language,* edited by T. Moore. New York: Academic Press, 1973.

CLARK, H. and S. HAVILAND, "Comprehension and the Given-New Contract," in *Discourse Production and Comprehension,* vol. 1. Edited by R. Freedle. Norwood, N.J.: Ablex, 1977, pp. 1–40.

COLE, P. and L. WOOD, "Differential Diagnosis," in *Pediatric Audiology,* edited by F. Martin. Englewood Cliffs, N.J.: Prentice-Hall, 1978.

DALE, P., *Language Development: Structure and Function,* 2nd ed. New York: Holt, Rinehart, and Winston, 1976.

DAVIS, B. and S. SEITZ, "Pronoun Assessment: A Free Speech Technique," *Journal of Speech and Hearing Research,* 18, (1975), 765–72.

DAWSON, M., "The Effect of Reinforcement and Verbal Rehearsal on Selective Attention in Learning Disabled Children," Doctoral Dissertation, 1978. *Dissertation Abstracts International,* 39, no. 7-2 (January 1979).

deVilliers, J. and P. deVilliers, *Language Acquisition.* Cambridge, Mass.: Harvard University Press, 1978.

Donahue, M., R. Pearl, and T. Bryan, "Learning Disabled Children's Conversational Competence: Responses to Inadequate Messages," *Applied Psycholinguistics,* 1, no. 4 (1980), 387–403.

Donaldson, M. and J. McGarrigle, "Some Clues to the Nature of Semantic Development," *Journal of Child Language,* 1, (1974), 185–94.

Dore, J., "A Pragmatic Description of Early Language Development," *The Journal of Psycholinguistic Research,* 3, no. 4 (1974), 343–50.

Dore, J., "Children's Illocutionary Acts," in *Discourse Production and Comprehension,* vol. 1, edited by R. Freedle. Norwood, N.J.: Ablex, 1977, pp. 227–44.

Dore, J., M. Gearhart, and D. Newman, "The Structure of Nursery School Conversations," *Children's Language,* vol. 1. Edited by K. Nelson, New York: Gardner Press, 1978, pp. 337–95.

Dunn, L., *Peabody Picture Vocabulary Test.* Circle Pines, Minn.: American Guidance Service, 1965.

Ervin-Tripp, S., "Wait for Me, Roller-Skate," in *Child Discourse,* edited by S. Ervin-Tripp and C. Mitchell-Kernan. New York: Academic Press, 1977.

Fey, M., L. Leonard, and K. Wilcox, "Speech Style Modifications of Language-Impaired Children," *Journal of Speech and Hearing Disorders,* 45, no. 1 (1981), 91–96.

Fielding, G. and C. Fraser, *Language and Interpersonal Relations, The Social Context of Language,* edited by I. Markova. New York: Wiley, 1978, pp. 217–32.

Fillmore, C., "The Case for Case," in *Universals in Linguistic Theory,* edited by E. Bach and R. Harms. New York: Holt, Rinehart, and Winston, 1968, pp. 1–88.

Foster, C., J. Gidden, and J. Stark, *Assessment of Children's Language Comprehension.* Palo Alto: Consulting Psychologists Press, 1972.

Gardner, H., M. Kircher, E. Winner, and D. Perkins, "Children's Metaphoric Productions and Preferences," *Journal of Child Language,* 2, (1975), 125–41.

Gardner, H., E. Winner, R. Bechhofer, and D. Wolf, "Figurative Language," in *Children's Language,* vol. 1. Edited by K. Nelson. New York: Gardner Press, 1978.

Garvey, C., "The Contingent Query: A Dependent Act in Conversation," in *Interaction, Conversation and the Development of Language,* edited by M. Lewis and L. Rosenblum. New York: Wiley, 1977, pp. 63–94.

Gentner, D., "Validation of a Related-Component Model of Verb Meaning," *Papers and Reports on Child Language,* 10, (1975), 69–79. California: Stanford University Department of Linguistics.

Goodman, Y., "Reading Comprehension: A Redundant Phase," in *Current Topics in Language: Introductory Readings,* edited by N. Johnson. Cambridge, Mass.: Winthrop, 1976, pp. 442–48.

Greenfield, P. and P. Zukow, "Psychogenesis of Presupposition," in *Children's Language,* vol. 1. Edited by K. Nelson. New York: Gardner Press, 1978.

Grice, H., "Logic and Conversation," in *Syntax and Semantics, vol. 3: Speech Acts,* edited by P. Cole and J. Morgan. New York: Academic Press, 1975.

GROSSFIELD, C. and E. GELLER, "Follow the Leader. Why Language Disordered Children Can't Be 'It,' " in *Working Papers in Experimental Speech, Language Pathology and Audiology,* vol. 9. New York: Department of Communication, Arts and Sciences, Queens College of the City University of New York, 1980.

HALL, P. and J. TOMBLIN, "A Follow-Up Study of Children with Articulation and Language Disorders," *Journal of Speech and Hearing Disorders,* 43, no. 2 (May 1978), 227–41.

HALLAHAN, D. and W. CRUICKSHANK, *Psychoeducational Foundations of Learning Disabilities.* Englewood Cliffs, N.J.: Prentice-Hall, 1973.

HALLAHAN, D., A. GAJAR, S. COHEN, and S. TARVER, "Selective Attention and Locus of Control in Learning Disabled and Normal Children," *Journal of Learning Disabilities,* 11, no. 4 (April 1978), 231–36.

HALLIDAY, M., *Explorations in the Functions of Language.* New York: Elsevier-North Holland Publishing, 1973.

HALLIDAY, M., *Learning How to Mean: Explanations in the Development of Language.* New York: Elsevier-North Holland Publishing, 1977.

HALLIDAY, M., *Language as Social Semiotic: The Social Interpretation of Language and Meaning.* London: University Park Press, 1978.

HASS, W. and J. WETTMAN, "Dimensions of Individual Difference in the Spoken Syntax of School Children," *Journal of Speech and Hearing Research,* 17, (1974), 455–69.

HORGAN, D., "Learning to Tell Jokes: A Case Study of Metalinguistic Abilities," *Journal of Child Language,* 8, no. 1 (February 1981), 217–24.

HYMES, D., "Introduction," in *Functions of Language in the Classrooms,* edited by C. Cazden, V. John, and D. Hymes. New York: Columbia University Teachers College Press, 1972.

JACKENDOFF, R., *Semantic Interpretation in Generative Grammar.* Cambridge, Mass.: MIT Press, 1972.

JACKSON, M., "Facilitating Reading Behavior in the Zero Reader," *Journal of Learning Disabilities,* 12, no. 3 (March 1979), 197–200.

JENKINS, J. and J. HELIOTIS, "Reading Comprehension Instruction: Findings from Behavioral and Cognitive Psychology," *Topics in Language Disorders,* 1, no. 2 (March 1981), 25–42. Edited by K. Butler and V. Brown. Rockville, Md.: Aspen Systems.

JOHNSON, D. and H. MYKLEBUST, *Learning Disabilities: Educational Principles and Practices.* New York: Grune and Stratton, 1967.

JOHNSON, M. and J. TOMBLIN, "The Reliability of Developmental Sentence Scoring as a Function of Sample Size," *Journal of Speech and Hearing Research,* 18, (1976), 372–80.

JOHNSON, N., "Summary: Language Acquisition and Teaching," in *Current Topics in Language: Introductory Readings,* edited by N. Johnson. Cambridge, Mass.: Winthrop, 1976, pp. 112–20.

JOHNSTON, J. and A. KAMHI, "The Same Can Be Less: Syntactic and Semantic Aspects of The Utterances of Language-Impaired Children," *Proceedings* from the First Wisconsin *Symposium on Research in Child Language Disorders,* Madison, Wis.: The University of Wisconsin, June, 1980, pp. 81–93.

JONES, N., "Non-Verbal Communication in Children," in *Non-Verbal Communication,* edited by R. Hinde. Cambridge, Mass.: Cambridge University Press, 1975, pp. 271–96.

JOOS, M., "The Style of the Five Clocks," in *Current Topics in Language: Introductory Readings,* edited by N. Johnson. Cambridge, Mass.: Winthrop, 1976, pp. 152–56.

KAIL, R. and C. MARSHALL, "Reading Skill and Memory Scanning," *Journal of Educational Psychology,* 70, (1978), 808–14.

KALGILL, M., F. FRIEDLAND, and R. SHAPIRO, "Predicting Learning Disabilities from Kindergarten Reports," *Journal of Learning Disabilities,* 6 (1973), 577–82.

KIRK, S., J. McCARTHY, and W. KIRK, *The Illinois Test of Psycholinguistic Abilities* rev. ed., Urbana, Ill.: University of Illinois Press, 1968.

KLASEN, E., *The Syndrome of Specific Dyslexia.* Baltimore: University Park Press, 1972.

KRAUSS, R., "Communication Models and Communication Behavior," in *Language Intervention from Ape to Child,* edited by R. Schiefelbusch and J. Hollis. Baltimore: University Park Press, 1979.

LEE, L., *Northwestern Syntax Screening Test.* Evanston, Ill.: Northwestern University Press, 1969.

LEE, L., *Developmental Sentence Analysis.* Evanston, Ill.: Northwestern University Press, 1974.

LEE, L., and S. CANTER, "Developmental Sentence Scoring: A Clinical Procedure for Estimating Syntactic Development in Children's Spontaneous Speech," *Journal of Speech and Hearing Disorders,* 36, (1971), 315–37.

LEONARD, L., "What Is Deviant Language?," *Journal of Speech and Hearing Disorders,* 37, (1972), 427–46.

LEONARD, L., C. PRUTTING, J. PEROZZI, and R. BERKLEY, "Nonstandardized Approaches to the Assessment of Language Behaviors," *Asha,* 20, (1978), 371–79.

LIBERMAN, I., "Segmentation of the Spoken Word and Reading Acquisition," Paper presented at the Symposium on Language and Perceptual Development. Philadelphia, March 31, 1973.

LIBERMAN, I., A. KIBERMAN, I. MATTINGLY, and D. SHANKWEILER, "Orthography and the Beginning Reader," in *Orthography, Reading, and Dyslexia,* edited by J. Kavanagh and R. Venezky. Baltimore: University Park Press, 1980.

LIBERMAN, I., D. SHANKWEILER, L. CAMP, B. HEIFETZ, and J. WERFELMAN, *Steps Toward Literacy.* A Report on Reading Prepared for the Working Group on Learning Failure and Unused Learning Potential for the President's Commission on Mental Health. Washington, D.C., November 1, 1977.

LOBAN, W., *The Language of Elementary School Children.* NCTE Research Report no. 1. Champaign, Ill.: National Center for Teachers of English, 1963.

LUCAS, E., The Behavioral Inventory of Speech Act Performances, in "The Feasability of Speech Acts as a Language Approach for Emotionally Disturbed Children," Doctoral Dissertation, University of Georgia, 1977. *Dissertation Abstracts International,* 1978.

LUCAS, E., *Semantic and Pragmatic Language Disorders: Assessment and Remediation.* Rockville, Md.: Aspen Systems, 1980.

MARSHALL, N., and M. GLOCK, "Comprehension of Connected Discourse: A Study into the Relationships Between the Structure of Texts and Information Recalled," *Reading Research Quarterly,* 13, no. 1 (1978–79), 10–56.

MATTINGLY, I., "Reading, The Linguistic Process, and Linguistic Awareness," in *Language by Ear and by Eye,* edited by J. Kavanagh and I. Mattingly. Cambridge, Mass.: MIT Press, 1972.

McNEILL, D., *The Acquisition of Language: The Study of Developmental Psycholinguistics.* New York: Harper and Row, 1970.

MECHAM, M., J. LOREN, and J. JONES, *Utah Test of Language Development* rev. ed. Salt Lake City: Communication Research Associates, 1967.

MENYUK, P., "Comparison of Grammar of Children with Functionally Deviant and Normal Speech," *Journal of Speech and Hearing Research,* 7, (1964), 109–21.

MENYUK, P., *Sentences Children Use.* Cambridge, Mass.: MIT Press, 1969.

MENYUK, P., and P. LOONEY, "Relationships among Components of the Grammar in Language Disorders," *Journal of Speech and Hearing Research,* 15, (1972), 395–406.

MILLER, J., *Assessing Language Production in Children.* Baltimore: University Park Press, 1981.

MILLER, J. and D. YODER, "On Developing the Content for the Language Teaching Program," *Mental Retardation,* (1972), 9–11.

MILLER, W., "The Language-Experience Approach to Reading," in *Current Topics in Language: Introductory Readings,* edited by N. Johnson. Cambridge Mass.: Winthrop, 1976, pp. 393–98.

MONROE, M., *Reading Aptitude Tests,* Primary Form. Boston: Houghton Mifflin, 1963.

MOREHEAD, D. and D. INGRAM, "The Development of Base Syntax in Normal and Linguistically Deviant Children," *Journal of Speech and Hearing Research,* 16, (1973), 331–52.

MUMA, J., *Language Handbook: Concepts, Assessments, Intervention.* Englewood Cliffs, N.J.: Prentice-Hall, 1978.

MURRAY, F. and J. PIKULSKY, *The Acquisition of Reading: Cognitive, Linguistic, and Perceptual Prerequisites.* Baltimore: University Park Press, 1978.

MYKLEBUST, H., *Development and Disorders of Written Language.* Vol. I. New York: Grune and Stratton, 1965.

MYKLEBUST, H., *Development and Disorders of Written Language.* Vol. II. New York: Grune and Stratton, 1973.

NELSON, N., "An Eclectic Model of Language Intervention for Disorders of Listening, Speaking, Reading, and Writing," *Topics in Language Disorders,* 1, no. 2 (March 1981), 1–24. Edited by K. Butler and V. Brown, Rockville, Md.: Aspen Systems.

NEWCOMER, P. and D. HAMMILL, *Test of Language Development.* Austin, Texas: Empiric Press, 1977.

OLSON, D., "Language Use for Communicating, Instructing and Thinking," in *Language Comprehension and the Acquisition of Knowledge*, edited by J. Carroll and R. Freedle. Washington, D.C.: V. H. Winston, 1972.

OLSON, D. and N. NICKERSON, "Language Development," in *Children's Language*, vol. 1. Edited by K. Nelson. New York: Gardner Press, 1978.

PAUL, L., "Social Language and Assembly Effects," Proceedings from the First Wisconsin *Symposium on Research in Child Language Disorders*. Madison: The University of Wisconsin, June, 1980, pp. 220–38.

PEARSON, D. and R. SPIRO, "Toward a Theory of Reading Comprehension Instruction," *Topics in Language Disorders*, 1, no. 1 (December 1980), 71–88. Edited by K. Butler and G. Wallach, Rockville, Md.: Aspen Systems.

PERFITTI, C. and A. LESGOLD, "Discourse Comprehension and Sources of Individual Differences," in Cognitive Processes in Comprehension, edited by M. Just and P. Carpenter. Hillsdale, N.J.: L. Erblaum Associates, 1977.

PRAEGER, E., S. BEECHER, M. STAFFORD, and E. WALLACE, *The Screening Test of Adolescent Language*. Seattle: University of Washington Press, 1980.

PRUTTING, C., C. GALLAGHER, and A. MULAC, "The Expressive Portion of the NSST Compared to the Spontaneous Language Sample," *Journal of Speech and Hearing Disorders*, 40, (1975), 40–48.

REES, N., "The Speech Pathologist and the Reading Process," *Asha*, 16, no. 55 (May 1974), 255–58.

REES, N., "Pragmatics of Language: Applications to Normal and Disordered Language Development," in *Bases of Language Intervention*, edited by R. Schiefelbusch. Baltimore: University Park Press, 1978, pp. 191–268.

REES, N. and SHULMAN, M., "I Don't Understand What You Mean by Comprehension," *Journal of Speech and Hearing Disorders*, 43, (1978), 208–19.

REID, D., "Child Reading: Readiness or Evolution?," *Topics in Language Disorders*, 1, no. 2 (March 1981), 61–72. Edited by K. Butler and V. Brown, Rockville, Md.: Aspen Systems.

RICHARDSON, S., "Foreward," in E. Wiig and E. Semel, *Language Disabilities in Children and Adolescents*. Columbus, Ohio: Charles E. Merrill, 1976, p. iii.

RIZZO, J. and M. STEPHENS, "Performance of Children with Normal and Impaired Oral Language Production on a Set of Auditory Comprehension Tests," *Journal of Speech and Hearing Disorders*, 46, no. 2 (May 1981), 150–59.

ROM, A. and L. BLISS, "A Comparison of Verbal Communicative Skills of Language Impaired and Normal Children," *Journal of Communication Disorders*, 14, no. 2 (1981), 133–40.

ROSENTHAL, D. and L. RESNICK, "Children's Solution Processes in Arithmetic Word Problems," *Journal of Educational Psychology*, 66 (1974), 817–25.

ROSENTHAL, J., "A Preliminary Psycholinguistic Study of Children with Learning Disabilities," *Journal of Learning Disabilities*, 3 (1970), 11–15.

ROTH, S. and C. PERFETTI, "A Framework for Reading, Language Comprehension, and Language Disability," *Topics in Language Disorders*, 1, no. 1 (December 1980), 29–46. Edited by K. Butler and G. Wallach, Rockville, Md.: Aspen Systems.

RUDEL, R., M. DENCKLA, and E. SPALTEN, "Paired Associate Learning of Morse Code and Braille Letter Names by Dyslexic and Normal Children," *Cortex*, 12, (1976), 61–70.

RUDER, K., "Planning and Programming for Language Intervention," in *Bases of Language Intervention*, edited by R. Schiefelbusch. Baltimore: University Park Press, 1978, pp. 320–71.

SACKS, H., E. SCHEGLOFF, and G. JEFFERSON, "A Simplest Systematics for the Organization of Turn-Taking in Conversation," *Language*, 50, (1974), 696–735.

SACHS, J. and J. DEVIN, "Young Children's Use of Age-Appropriate Speech Styles in Social Interaction and Role-Playing," *Journal of Child Language*, 3, (1976), 81–98.

SAWYER, J. and S. LIPA, "The Route to Reading: A Perspective," *Topics in Language Disorders*, 1, no. 2 (March 1981), 43–60. Edited by K. Butler and V. Brown, Rockville, Md.: Aspen Systems.

SCHATZ, M. and R. GELMAN, "The Development of Communication Skills; Modifications in the Speech of Young Children as a Function of the Listeners," *Monographs of the Society for Research in Child Development*, 38, (1973), 1–36.

SCHLESINGER, I., *Sentence Structure and the Reading Process*. The Hague: Mouton, 1968.

SEARLE, J., *Speech Acts: An Essay in the Philosophy of Language*. London: Cambridge University Press, 1976.

SEMEL, E. and E. WIIG, "Comprehension of Syntactic Structures and Critical Verbal Elements by Children with Learning Disabilities," *Journal of Learning Disabilities*, 8 (1975), 53–58.

SEMEL, E. and E. WIIG, *Clinical Evaluation of Language Function*. Columbus, Ohio: Charles E. Merrill, 1980.

SHANKWEILER, D. and I. LIBERMAN, " 'Misreading' A Search for Cues," in *Language by Ear and by Eye*, edited by J. Kavanagh and I. Mattingly. Cambridge, Mass.: MIT Press, 1972.

SHERIDAN, M. and C. PECKHAM, "Follow-up to Sixteen Years of School Children Who Had Marked Speech Defects at Seven Years," *Child Care, Health and Development*, 4, no. 3, (May–June, 1978), 145–57.

SHRINER, T., "A Review of Mean Length of Response as a Measure of Expressive Language Development in Children," *Journal of Speech and Hearing Disorders*, 14, (1969), 61–67.

SIEGEL, G. and J. SPRADLIN, "Programming for Language and Communication Therapy," in *Language Intervention Strategies*, edited by R. Schiefelbusch. Baltimore: University Park Press, 1978, pp. 357–98.

SILVERMAN, R., N. ZIGMOND, J. ZIMMERMAN, A. VALLERCORSA, "Improving Written Expression in Learning Disabled Students," *Topics in Language Disorders*, 1, no. 2 (March 1981), 91–99. Edited by K. Butler and V. Brown, Rockville, Md.: Aspen Systems.

SIMON, C., *Communicative Competence: A Functional-Pragmatic Approach to Language Therapy*. Tucson, Ariz.: Communication Skill Builders, 1979.

SLOBIN, D., *Psycholinguistics*. Glenview, Ill.: Scott, Foresman, 1971.

SMILEY, S., D. OAKLEY, D. WORTHEN, J. CAMPIONE, and A. BROWN, "Recall of Thematically Relevant Material by Adolescent Good and Poor Readers as a Function Versus Oral Presentation," *Journal of Educational Psychology*, 69, (1977), 381–87.

SNYDER, L., "Have We Prepared the Language Disordered Child for School?," *Topics in Language Disorders*, 1, no. 1 (December 1980), 29–46. Edited by K. Butler and G. Wallach, Rockville, Md.: Aspen Systems.

STARK, J. and G. WALLACH, "The Path to a Concept of Language Learning Disabilities," *Topics in Language Disorders*, 1, no. 1 (December 1980), 1–15. Edited by K. Butler and G. Wallach, Rockville, Md.: Aspen Systems.

STEPHENS, M., *Stephens Oral Language Screening Test.* Peninsula, Ohio: Intermin Publishers, 1977.

SWANSON, L., "Verbal Encoding Effects on the Visual Short-Term Memory of Learning-Disabled and Normal Readers," *Journal of Educational Psychology*, 70, no. 4 (August 1968), 539–44.

TEMPLIN, M., "Certain Language Skills in Children: Their Development and Interrelationships," *Child Welfare Monograph No. 126*, Minneapolis: University of Minnesota Press, 1957.

TERMAN, L. and M. MERRILL, *Stanford-Binet Intelligence Scale.* Boston: Houghton Mifflin, 1969.

TORONTO A., *Toronto Tests of Receptive Vocabulary (English/Spanish).* Austin, Texas: Academic Tests, 1977.

TOUGH, J., *The Development of Meaning.* New York: Halsted Press, 1977.

TRANTHAM, C. and J. PEDERSEN, *Normal Language Development: The Key to Diagnosis and Therapy for Language-Disordered Children.* Baltimore: Williams and Wilkins, 1976.

TRAVIS, L., ed., *Handbook of Speech Pathology.* New York: Appleton-Century-Crofts, 1957.

TYACK, D., "The Use of Language Samples in a Clinical Setting," *Journal of Learning Disabilities*, 6, (1972), 213–16.

U. S. OFFICE OF EDUCATION, "Assistance to States for Education of Handicapped Children: Procedures for Evaluating Specific Learning Disabilities," *Federal Register*, 1977, 65082–65085.

VAN RIPER, C., *Speech Correction: Principles and Methods.* Englewood Cliffs, N.J.: Prentice-Hall, 1962.

VELLUTINO, F., "Toward an Understanding of Dyslexia: Psychological Factors in Specific Reading Dyslexia," in *Dyslexia: An Appraisal of Current Knowledge*, edited by P. Benton and D. Pearl. New York: Oxford University Press, 1978, pp. 63–111.

VELLUTINO, F., "The Validity of Perceptual Deficit Explanations of Reading Disability: A Reply to Fletcher and Satz," *Journal of Learning Disabilities*, 12, no. 3 (March 1979), 160–167.

VENEZKY, R., "Spelling-to-Sound Correspondences," in *Communicating by Language: The Reading Process*, edited by J. Kavanagh. Bethesda, Md.: U.S. Department of Health, Education and Welfare, National Institutes of Health, 1968.

Vogel, S., "Syntactic Abilities in Normal and Dyslexic Children," *Journal of Learning Disabilities,* 7, (1974), 103–9.

Vygotsky, L., *Thought and Language.* Cambridge, Mass.: MIT Press, 1962.

Wallach, G. and **D. Lee,** "So You Want to Know What to Do with Language Disabled Children Above the Age of Six," *Topics in Language Disorders,* 1, no. 1 (December 1980), 99–113. Edited by K. Butler and G. Wallach, Rockville, Md.: Aspen Systems.

Wechsler, D., *Manual for the Wechsler Intelligence Scale for Children.* New York: Psychological Corporation, 1949.

Weiner, E., "Diagnostic Evaluation of Written Skills," *Journal of Learning Disabilities,* 13, (1980), 48–53.

Weiner, P., "A Language Delayed Child at Adolescence," *Journal of Speech and Hearing Disorders,* 39, (1974), 202–12.

Wiig, E. and **E. Semel,** "Productive Language Abilities in Learning Disabled Adolescents," *Journal of Learning Disabilities,* 8, (1975), 578–86.

Wiig, E. and **E. Semel,** *Language Disabilities in Children and Adolescents.* Columbus, Ohio: Charles Merrill, 1976.

Wiig, E. and **E. Semel,** *Language Assessment and Intervention for the Learning Disabled.* Columbus, Ohio: Charles Merrill, 1980.

Winitz, H., "The Development of Speech and Language in the Normal Child," in *Speech Pathology*, edited by R. Reiber and R. Brubaker. Philadelphia: J. B. Lippincott Co., 1966, pp. 42–76.

Winner, E., A. Rosentiel, and **H. Gardner,** "The Development of Metaphoric Understanding," *Developmental Psychology,* 12, (1976), 289–97.

Wolski, W., *The Michigan Picture Language Inventory.* Ann Arbor, Mich.: University of Michigan Press, 1962.

Wood, L., *An Analysis of Selected Morphemes in the Spontaneous Speech of Normal and Language-Impaired Children.* Doctoral Dissertation, The University of Texas at Austin, 1976.

Yassi, R., "Contributions to the Speech-Language Specialist for Prescriptive Teaching," *Deveureaux Forum,* 13, (Winter 1978), 16–18.

Zigmond, N., A. Vallecorsa, and **G. Leinhardt,** "Reading Instruction for Students with Learning Disabilities," *Topics in Language Disorders,* 1, no. 1 (December 1980), 89–98. Edited by K. Butler and G. Wallach, Rockville, Md.: Aspen Systems.

DATE DUE			
NOV 1 '93			
MAR 16 '94			
MAR 14 '95			
MAR 14 '95			
FEB 0 2 1998			
NOV 2 7 2000			